Developmental Perspectives on Teaching and Learning Thinking Skills

Contributions to Human Development

Vol. 21

Series Editor
Deanna Kuhn, New York, N.Y.

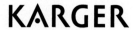

Basel · München · Paris · London · New York · New Delhi · Bangkok · Singapore · Tokyo · Sydney

Developmental Perspectives on Teaching and Learning Thinking Skills

Volume Editor
Deanna Kuhn, New York, N.Y.

2 figures and 3 tables, 1990

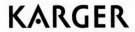

Basel · München · Paris · London · New York · New Delhi · Bangkok · Singapore · Tokyo · Sydney

Contributions to Human Development

Library of Congress Cataloging-in-Publication Data
Developmental perspectives on teaching and learning thinking skills /
volume editor, Deanna Kuhn.
(Contributions to human development; v. 21)
Includes bibliographical references and index.
1. Thought and thinking – Study and teaching.   2. Cognition in children.
I. Kuhn, Deanna.   II. Series.
LB1590.3.D49   1990
370.15'2 – dc20
ISBN 3–8055–5205–X

©   Copyright 1990 by S. Karger AG, P.O. Box, CH– 4009 Basel (Switzerland)
Printed in Switzerland by Thür AG Offsettdruck, Pratteln
ISBN 3–8055–5205–X

Contents

Contents

K.S. Kitchener, K.W. Fischer

A Skill Approach to the Development of Reflective Thinking

L. Okagaki, R.J. Sternberg

Teaching Thinking Skills: We're Getting the Context Wrong

M. Krechevsky, H. Gardner

Approaching School Intelligently: An Infusion Approach

W. Damon

Social Relations and Children's Thinking Skills

Contents

A.L. Brown, J.C. Campione
Communities of Learning and Thinking, or a Context by Any Other Name

Contributors

Baron, Jonathan, Department of Psychology, University of Pennsylvania,
Philadelphia, PA 19104-6196 (USA)

Brown, Ann L., Education in Math, Science and Technology, Tolman Hall,
School of Education, University of California, Berkeley, CA 94720 (USA)

Campione, Joseph C., Education in Math, Science and Technology, Tolman Hall,
School of Education, University of California, Berkeley, CA 94720 (USA)

Damon, William, Department of Education, Brown University,
Providence, RI 02912 (USA)

Fischer, Kurt W., Department of Human Development, Graduate School of Education,
Harvard University, Cambridge, MA 02138 (USA)

Gardner, Howard, Harvard Project Zero, Graduate School of Education,
Harvard University, Cambridge, MA 02138 (USA)

Glaser, Robert, Learning Research and Development Center, University of Pittsburgh,
Pittsburgh, PA 15260 (USA)

Kitchener, Karen Strohm, School of Education, University of Denver,
Denver, CO 80208 (USA)

Krechevsky, Mara, Harvard Project Zero, Graduate School of Education,
Harvard University, Cambridge, MA 02138 (USA)

Kuhn, Deanna, Teachers College, Columbia University, PO Box 119,
New York, NY 10027 (USA)

Okagaki, Lynn, Department of Psychology, Yale University, PO Box 11A Yale Station,
New Haven, CT 06515 (USA)

Schauble, Leona, Learning Research and Development Center, University of Pittsburgh,
Pittsburgh, PA 15260 (USA)

Sternberg, Robert J., Department of Psychology, Yale University, PO Box 11A,
Yale Station, New Haven, CT 06515 (USA)

Kuhn D (ed): Developmental Perspectives on Teaching and Learning Thinking Skills.
Contrib Hum Dev. Basel, Karger, 1990, vol 21, pp 1–8

Introduction

Deanna Kuhn

The concern that schools are not doing what they should to educate our youth has never been greater. While some of this concern is focused on students' lack of knowledge in basic subject matter areas of science, mathematics, social studies, and literature, of even greater and increasing concern is the fact that students who progress through our school systems seem not to have acquired the ability to think well. They exhibit at best weak ability to consider alternatives and weigh evidence, reaching independent judgments that they are able to justify in a reasoned way. These are abilities clearly requisite to participation in a rational society, and, arguably, to a fulfilled individual life as well.

Educators over the last decade have shown tremendous interest and investment in developing new curricula, and reforming existing curricula, to promote the development of thinking skills. We would expect these efforts on the part of educators to be supported and enriched by a knowledge base provided by researchers in cognitive and developmental psychology regarding the nature of thinking and its development. The premise underlying the present volume is that in general educators have not had the benefit of this support to the extent they might or should have. The reasons that this has been so I have speculated about previously [Kuhn, 1989a]. Some likely reasons include (a) the tendency of cognitive and developmental researchers until recently to study thinking in forms and contexts removed from those that occur in school or everyday activities, and (b) a focus on the products rather than the process of thinking and knowing. Other trends more specific to developmental psychology of the last decade, but having a similar effect, are (c) a focus on the organization of knowledge within specific knowledge domains, rather than forms of thinking that extend across domains, and (d) emphasis on identification of cognitive competencies in their earliest, most implicit forms, rather than the explicit forms of knowing of concern to educators.

The focus of the present volume, however, is a forward-looking one, emphasizing the fact that this situation has clearly begun to change. The following chapters all illustrate that those who wish to promote the acquisition of thinking skills can and should benefit from the knowledge and understanding that researchers in cognitive and developmental psychology have achieved. In this introduction I identify five broad respects in which current psychological research provides fundamental insight into teaching and learning thinking skills. Each of the five is well reflected in the chapters that follow.

Identifying and Analyzing Thinking Skills

The first and clearly most fundamental kind of knowledge that psychological research stands to provide is the identification and analysis of thinking skills. Educational programs typically have based their efforts on one or another intuitively-based taxonomy of thinking skills, with little theoretical or empirical justification of why it is this specific set of skills that should be the object of educational efforts. To justify their implementation, on even an experimental basis, thinking skill programs should be informed by psychological knowledge regarding the nature of the thinking strategies that underlie both the faulty and sound thinking that people are observed to use.

Researchers traditionally have not focused their investigations on the actual thinking that takes place in school and other natural contexts, as I noted above, and hence they have had little to offer in the way of theoretical or empirical analysis of thinking skills people might be observed to use outside of artificial problem contexts devised for research purposes. This situation has changed dramatically in recent years, however, and there now exists fundamental knowledge of both a theoretical and empirical nature that is of direct relevance to teaching thinking. Cognitive psychologists have contributed a growing body of work on the nature of informal reasoning [Voss et al., in press] that tells us much about the good and poor reasoning that occurs in the thinking people do about real-life, important problems, typically ones that lack simple solutions. Also from modern cognitive psychology comes the conceptual perspective and research pertaining to judgment and decision [Baron, 1985; Kahneman, Slovic, and Tversky, 1982]. This work has had very little impact on thinking skills efforts, and Baron's chapter in this volume well establishes its relevance. What thinking errors do people in fact make commonly? Unless good and faulty thinking are defined in precise, empirically-grounded ways, Baron observes, teaching efforts risk fixing what's not broken.

Developmental psychologists likewise increasingly have turned their attention to situations more like those in which thinking occurs naturally. They have identified not only a range of good and faulty thinking strategies, but also critical information about the course of development of these strategies across the life span. The chapter by Schauble and Glaser in this volume well represents this growing body of knowledge. Schauble and Glaser focus on comparisons of the thinking of elementary school children and adults as they interpret the bearing of new evidence on their existing understandings of how complex multivariable phenomena operate. Their findings converge with those from several other laboratories in establishing that children and adults differ in more than the extent and organization of the knowledge they possess. They differ as well in the thinking strategies they bring to bear in coordinating their existing knowledge with new evidence and revising their beliefs, i.e., in the *process* in terms of which their knowledge is expanded and reorganized [Dunbar and Klahr, 1988; Kuhn, 1989b; Schauble, 1990]. In his chapter, Baron raises the possibility that some thinking errors may become more prevalent with age. In either case – whether changes are progressive or regressive – educational interventions to teach thinking strategies clearly must base their efforts on a thorough understanding of the changes these strategies normally undergo over the life span in the absence of such intervention.

The thinking skills identified and examined by the present authors by no means comprise an exhaustive set. Indeed, the definitional task is an ongoing one, as empirical findings refine conceptualizations which in turn generate new investigations. Though the thrust of their work has to do with the processes by means of which thinking skills are facilitated, in their chapter Brown and Campione perform the important service of expanding our conceptions of what thinking skills include, by reconceptualizing the traditional domain of reading as one in which thinking skills figure prominently.

Identification and analysis of the thinking strategies involved in both sound and faulty thinking are clearly the 'meat and potatoes' that provide a sound base for educational efforts to teach thinking. As the present chapters make clear, the research task extends beyond identification of thinking skills themselves. Equally important, how do they interrrlate? To what degrees are they tied to certain kinds of content? And also of fundamental importance, what course of development do they show naturally? As Kitchener and Fischer stress in their chapter, thinking skills are not simply isolated techniques or bits of procedural knowledge to be passed on from instructor to student in an accumulative fashion. Thinking has organization, coherence, and certain developmental directions, all of which must be well understood by those who wish to facilitate it.

Yet, the chapters in this volume reflect not only the essential foundation that research provides in understanding the nature of thinking skills and their development. They also demonstrate ways in which research can enrich and expand conceptions of additional factors that come into play in teaching and learning thinking skills. Such factors, highlighted by several of the present chapters, bear crucially on the outcome of educational efforts.

Examining the Understanding of Thinking

One additional factor, beyond thinking skills themselves, that research on thinking points to as critically important is people's understanding of thinking. As Kitchener and Fischer emphasize, thinking strategies are interrelated and organized into a system that represents the individual's mode of understanding the world. This system includes understanding of thinking itself. Such understanding may pertain to a particular strategy – when is it appropriately used and what does it buy one? Krechevsky and Gardner provide a number of such examples in their chapter, as does Baron. It is this understanding that weighs heavily in the issue that educators already have discovered as critical – will newly learned strategies transfer to new contexts beyond the one in which they were acquired?

Another, broader kind of understanding is of the nature of thinking and knowledge more generally. It is the development of this understanding that Kitchener and Fischer address in their chapter. Like the development of thinking itself, this understanding progressees in an organized, rather than haphazard, fashion. The details of the sequence described vary, but research from a number of independent sources, originating with Perry [1970], points to a similar progression in the epistemological understanding of processes of thinking and knowing [Kitchener and King, 1990; Kuhn, forthcoming]. Individuals initially believe that even complex judgments about difficult issues can be made with certainty, given sufficient information or expertise. Many subsequently shift from this absolutist stance to a relativist one in which nothing is known for certain, as all knowledge depends on the personal, subjective perspective of individuals, who often disagree; as a result, all perspectives on a problem are equally valid. Only later is the acceptance of uncertainty integrated with the recognition that multiple perspectives or judgments are nevertheless subjectable to a process of inquiry and evaluation that can show some to be more correct than others. Even though all of the research shows them to be a minority, it is only individuals whose epistemological understanding is of the latter sort for whom the skills of thinking assume real significance. It is only for them that knowing is the product of a process of reasoned argument. It is as important, then, for educators to promote progress toward this evaluative conception of thinking and knowing as it is to foster the thinking skills that are necessary to practice it.

The Determining Role of Context

A third kind of knowledge that research on thinking provides is the crucial relevance of the environmental contexts in which thinking takes place. Their role is examined in the chapter by Okagaki and Sternberg. Certain contexts elicit and reward certain kinds of thinking. Hence, it is not enough to teach a set of thinking skills without the learner's understanding the relations between these skills and the cognitive and social demands of the various environmental contexts that make up the learner's sphere of experience. To do so is to expend the effort of both teacher and learner to learn skills with no sense of whether the learner will ever have occasion to use them. As both the chapters by Okagaki and Sternberg and by Krechevsky and Gardner emphasize, the school context, though a common one, is a very specialized context. It calls for metacognitive understanding of the specialized forms of thinking that it promotes, and, as Okagaki and Sternberg show, transfer from school to non-school contexts may be especially difficult.

Thinking as a Social Activity

A fourth kind of knowledge provided by research on thinking also has to do with context. It highlights the fact that the contexts in which teaching and learning thinking skills occur are most often social ones. The idea that social factors affect cognitive functioning is a familiar one. Less common is the proposal made both by Damon in his chapter and by Brown and Campione in theirs that thinking processes may themselves reflect the social activities in which the thinker engages. As Damon phrases it, over the course of development 'children's thinking tends to replicate the procedural logic of the social communications in which they participate'. This is a very productive idea if taken seriously, for in addition to linking the interpersonal and individual planes, as Damon notes, it suggests a way to externalize the internal thinking strategies we would like to foster within the individual, both for the research objective of analysis and the practical objective of facilitation. The correspondence between mental and social activities is perhaps easiest to see among young children and the parent or teacher who guides their developing skill, and it is here that it has most often been explored. But, increasingly, it is being recognized that the correspondence is fully as rich and productive to examine in the case of more complex cognitive skills shown by older children, as Damon's and Brown and Campione's chapters document, and even in the argumentive reasoning central to what we regard as critical thinking among adolescents and adults [Kuhn, forthcoming].

The Development of Thinking Skills

The conception of thinking as a social activity suggests but does not dictate a model of how thinking skills develop. Many social-cognitive theorists lean toward a Vygotskian [1978] model in which cognition expressed in social forms is interiorized as individual thought, while others would favor the more Piagetian view of parallel, but coordinated, development on the individual and social planes [Piaget, 1950]. The question of process brings us finally to a fifth kind of knowledge that research on thinking stands to contribute, one as fundamental as the kind described first, devoted to identifying thinking skills, and that is understanding of the process by means of which thinking skills develop.

Because specific educational influences interact in often complex ways with developmental change that is occurring as a result of more general forms of experience, the study of process is a difficult one, but researchers are increasingly coming to agree that the method must be a microgenetic one in which the change process is observed over an extended period of time. The chapters by Schauble and Glaser and by Brown and Campione illustrate such approaches. Whether thinking skills can be taught explicitly or must be constructed by learners themselves through their own activities, a contrast that Damon probes, is unresolved. What the social perspective discussed above makes clear, however, is that in any successful learning context the relationship between teacher and learner must be a collaborative one. Therefore, what the learners themselves contribute to the interaction must continually be attended to. Significantly, many of the questions that researchers debate are the same ones that concern educators: Should teaching be implicit and practice-based or explicit? Should it occur in the context of or distinct from academic subject matter? The fact that several of the present authors have devised their own experimental programs to explore these questions and others testifies to the integral relations that must exist between research and practice in the teaching and learning of thinking skills – a set of close and productive relations that the present volume shows are increasingly coming to be realized.

Defining Educational Goals

In concluding, it is worth noting that the researchers who seek to enhance our understanding of thinking and its development are collaborating with educators in what is likely the most significant educational enterprise of all – defining the objectives we wish education to accomplish. The traditional role of psychologist collaborating with the educator has been one of psychologist as technologist, advising the educator regarding how to achieve curriculum objectives, once these objectives have been stipulated by the educator. If the educator's objectives are identified as the mastery of thinking skills, the psychologist might assist by developing instructional methods or by designing research to evaluate outcomes. But in the latter task we encouter a paradox, for often the criterion of success in such evaluations has been improved school performance, whether or not achievement in school involves the skills that are promoted by the thinking skills curriculum being evaluated.

The direction of this relationship arguably should be the reverse. Rather than the success of the thinking skills program being measured by existing school curriculum, the nature of the thinking skills identified as important to effective thinking should shape the content of the school curriculum. In this case, the researcher's role becomes central, shifting from implementer to definer of educational goals. To further clarify and delineate the nature of the thinking competencies that we want education to impart to our youth is an enterprise that both researchers and educators can involve themselves in, with the knowledge that no educational endeavor is of greater importance to education as a field or to our society's future.

References

Baron, J. (1985). *Rationality and intelligence.* New York: Cambridge University Press.

Dunbar, K., & Klahr, D. (1988). Developmental differences in scientific discovery strategies. In D. Klahr & K. Kotovsky (Eds.), *Complex information processing: The impace of Herbert A. Simon* (Proceedings of the 21st Carnegie-Mellon Symposium on Cognition, pp. 104–144). Hillsdale NJ: Erlbaum.

Kahneman, D., Slovic, P., & Tversky, A. (Eds.). (1982). *Judgment under uncertainty: Heuristics and biases.* New York: Cambridge University Press.

Kitchener, K.S., & King, P.M. (1990). The reflective judgment model: Ten years of research. In M.L. Commons, C. Armon, L. Kohlberg, F.A. Richards, T.A. Grotzer, & J.D. Sinnott (Eds.), *Adult development 3: Models and methods in the study of adolescent and adult thought.* New York: Praeger.

Kuhn, D. (1989a). Making cognitive development research relevant to education. In W. Damon (Ed.), *Child development today and tomorrow.* San Francisco: Jossey-Bass.

Kuhn, D. (1989b). Children and adults as intuitive scientists. *Psychological Review, 96,* 674–689.

Kuhn, D. (forthcoming). *The skills of argument.*

Perry, W. (1970). *Forms of intellectual and ethical development in the college years.* New York: Holt, Rinehart & Winston.

Piaget, J. (1950). *The psychology of intelligence.* London: Routledge & Kegan Paul.

Schauble, L. (1990). Belief revision in children: The role of prior knowledge and strategies for generating evidence. *Journal of Experimental Child Psychology, 49,* 31–57.

Vygotsky, L.S. (1978). *Mind in society: The development of higher psychological processes.* Cambridge MA: Harvard University Press.

Voss, J., Perkins, D., & Segal, J. (in press). *Informal reasoning and education.* Hillsdale NJ: Erlbaum.

Kuhn D (ed): Developmental Perspectives on Teaching and Learning Thinking Skills.
Contrib Hum Dev. Basel, Karger, 1990, vol 21, pp 9–27

Scientific Thinking in Children and Adults

Leona Schauble, Robert Glaser

Education has always been concerned with cultivating abilities to reason. Aiding students to use their minds better has been an essential aspi-
ration of teaching. Yet, we see too many apparently educated people who
do not use their knowledge well. Knowing is only part of being educated;
thinking and reasoning with what we know completes it. We can ask, however, whether it is really necessary to teach thinking and reasoning. People
do reason spontaneously without being taught to do so. Every day we analyze and generalize, make analogies, deduce and induce, form and test
ideas and hypotheses, and solve problems. Children do these things long
before they encounter formal schooling, and adults make numerous complex decisions in the course of their daily lives. But observation and
research have documented our limitations as thinkers and problem solvers
and the ways in which our reasoning commonly goes astray [Halpern,
1984; Nickerson et al., 1985]. At present, there is a demand for making
opportunities for thinking and reasoning more prevalent in the actual
teaching of school subjects. There is concern that schooling, with its
emphasis on curriculum coverage and didactic instruction, does not
presently maximize opportunities for thinking.

As a consequence, among educators, teaching higher-order thinking
skills has become the slogan of the day [Chipman et al., 1985; Glaser, 1985;
Nickerson et al., 1985; Segal et al., 1985; Resnick, 1987]. However, current
research on thinking skills poses a dilemma between placing instructional
emphasis on general, domain-independent skills and domain-specific skills
and knowledge. In science education, this dilemma plays itself out in debates
concerning the relative value of 'process' approaches to teaching science
versus emphasis on building large, well-structured bodies of content knowledge that enable problem solving. Educators on one side of this debate argue

that the rapid proliferation of new information in science and technology requires an instructional focus on the fostering of general skills that will presumably then be available to support the learning of new information. Others counter that when knowledgeable people solve problems, they make use of patterns of organized knowledge that enable them to minimize or bypass less efficient general processes. General problem-solving skills may be more involved in novel or unfamiliar domains. Thus, it is claimed that both levels of thinking can be taught, as subject-matter knowledge and skill are acquired. These debates are unproductive, however, in the absence of a well-grounded understanding of the kinds of proficient reasoning we want our students to achieve in various domains of knowledge and of the strengths and weaknesses characteristic of their reasoning. Furthermore, discussions concerning how to develop curricula and programs for teaching scientific reasoning need to be informed by empirical research that closely analyzes the cognitive processes and structures of knowledge actually employed when people reason in school subjects like science.

In this chapter we describe a program of research on scientific thinking skills in contexts of self-directed experimentation. Children and adults negotiate the cycle of developing hypotheses, designing experiments to test those hypotheses, managing and interpreting the data they generate, making inferences on the basis of these data, and revising their hypotheses. The individuals studied typically have some beginning conceptions in the domain they are working in, and are observed as they plan and carry out a program of inquiry to expand or revise their current knowledge. Until very recently, psychological research has focused on domain-general strategic components of scientific thinking such as hypothesis formation [Bruner et al., 1956; Simon and Kotovsky, 1963], experimental design [Karmiloff-Smith and Inhelder, 1974; Kuhn and Phelps, 1982; Siegler and Liebert, 1975], and the interpretation of evidence [Einhorn and Hogarth, 1986; Mynatt et al., 1977; Robinson and Hastie, 1985]. In these investigations, for the most part, the influence of domain knowledge was not a variable of interest. However, as Klahr and Dunbar [1988] have suggested, it is unlikely that experimentation strategies are ever uncontaminated by the influence of knowledge or ideas about the domain being explored; and conversely, the activity of experimenting presumes the purpose of revising or extending one's domain knowledge or understanding. In their research, prior beliefs were found to be influential in determining the hypotheses that subjects generated, the experiments they conducted and the inferences they made.

The work discussed here continues along this line of studying scientific reasoning about knowledge domains rich enough so that prior beliefs significantly influence the reasoning process. We also continue a recent trend of investigating larger, coherent episodes of reasoning that occur over an extended period of time and that include the full cycle of hypothesis generation, experimentation, data interpretation, and hypothesis revision. Some of the studies [Schauble, 1990] have been conducted with children, and others [Glaser et al., 1988; Shute et al., 1989] with adults. Although these studies were not explicitly designed to compare children and adults, in this chapter we describe similarities and differences in the scientific thinking they display.

In our studies, computer-based laboratories serve both as the main stimuli for the studies and as data-collection instruments. The laboratories provide subjects the opportunity to perform experiments in a simulated domain that behaves in important ways like the real world. Our circuit laboratory, *Voltaville,* simulates the behavior of d.c. circuits and circuit components; *Refract* simulates the domain of geometrical optics; *Smithtown* simulates the laws of microeconomics in a hypothetical town; and, finally, *Daytona,* a microworld of race cars, incorporates causal relations among car design features and speed. The laboratories allow users to design experiments, make predictions, interpret outcomes, manage data, and record results. Subjects work with one or more computer laboratories over several sessions, with the general objective of learning which variables are relevant and then discovering the laws and principles specifying the relations of the relevant variables.

We begin by describing a group of preadolescent children who explored the computer microworld of race cars. We then compare adult subjects working for a shorter period with the same microworld. Finally, we examine the behavior of adults working with the more complex laboratories indicated above.

Children's Exploration of the Race Cars Microworld

It is at around 10 years of age that children begin to show certain skills in generating and interpreting experiments, such as setting up comparisons in which only one variable is varied and correctly interpreting patterns of data indicating that there is no causal relation between a variable and an outcome [Kuhn et al., 1988; Tschirgi, 1980]. In our study [Schauble, 1990], fifth- and sixth-grade children (10–12 years old), for seven weekly 30 min sessions engaged in self-directed exploration of Daytona, the microworld of race cars, a domain in which children had some familiarity and beliefs but were not experts. The microworld was designed to be complex enough so that children found it challenging over the seven-week period, but simple enough so they could construct at least some understanding of the causal relations that existed. Experiments could be set up by constructing race cars from five different design features; each experiment could include up to three cars at a time. The subject then 'drove' the cars on the computer screen, producing an outcome of the experiment. Subjects were encouraged to keep records in 'logbooks' that were provided.

Three of the five design features had a causal relation to speed. Of these, two (engine size and the tailfin) had an interacting effect (cars without tailfins were faster, but only on cars with large engines). The third (wheel size) had a nonlinear relation to speed (cars with large or small wheels went the same speed and slower than cars with medium-sized wheels). The two remaining features (color and muffler) had no causal effects. Each appropriate change in a causal feature changed the speed of a car by one unit; that is, the car would travel one more unit of distance (marked by numbered flags) within a constant time period. Car features were configured to the theories that children of this age typically held (explored earlier with an independent group of children). Most children believed that the engine size and muffler would affect the speed of a car and that the tailfin and the color would have no effect. Most children believed that wheel size would be causal, but some thought small wheels would be fastest, and others felt large wheels would be fastest. Thus, some of the effects were congruent with children's prior beliefs, while others were discrepant. Consequently, the microworld provided many opportunities for both causal and noncausal theories to be confirmed and disconfirmed.

Children appeared to make considerable progress in coming to understand this microworld, even though they did so in ways that looked rather haphazard. Most of the 22 children succeeded in correctly identifying most of the simple causal features, although they had more success with those features that confirmed their prior beliefs than with the disconfirming features. Only 2 of the 22 discovered the interaction between tailfin and engine. Children made steady improvement in their ability to accurately predict the speed of any individual car, showing change in their theories about the effects of the design features and the way these features acted together.

When we turn to examining *how* the children achieved this progress, however, the picture is not one of steady improvement. Children appeared to proceed not by using sound strategies for designing and interpreting experiments. Children typically attended to only a small percentage of the available information (i.e., they constructed a mean of only 53% of the possible 48 cars and frequently constructed the same cars over and over). They appeared not to have a clear idea of the possible variation (most children estimated the maximum number of unique cars that could be built to be around 12). Furthermore, children typically did not come to a conclusion about a feature and stick to it. Instead, they changed their minds, sometimes with surprising frequency. Their judgments vacillated especially frequently about those features that worked in ways inconsistent with their original beliefs.

Generation of Evidence

Examination of the experimentation strategies children used indicates characteristic weaknesses as well. About two-thirds of the time, children designed experiments that did not support a definitive conclusion. Typically, they constructed cars including variations of several features and then tried to make inferences about the effects of a single feature. Or they might construct only one car and draw a conclusion about a feature on this basis – for example, building a car with a large engine and then concluding that 'Engine makes a difference, because this car had a big engine and it went fast'. (Another kind of invalid experiment involved constructing three cars with large engines and coming to the identical conclusion.)

Interpretation of Evidence

Children appeared quite content to make inferences based on these invalid data. As a result, two thirds of their judgments were invalid, that is, either incorrect or based on inconclusive evidence. Only in about 10% of their experiments did they note that they could not interpret the evidence, although 66% of their experiments did not support a definitive conclusion. These invalid judgments served to preserve their incorrect prior beliefs or to resurrect incorrect prior beliefs that they had earlier disconfirmed. Finally, 25% of their justifications were based not on their experiments, but on their beliefs about cars. In these cases, only after being prompted by the experimenter ('But what do these roadtests tell you about the cars?'), did children attend to the evidence at all.

Data Management

Children rarely used their logbooks, either to work out plans or to record experiments; instead, they preferred to rely on memory to recall what they had done from session to session. No child consistently recorded information about the covariation of features and outcomes (4 children did so inconsistently); nor did children make systematic use of the records automatically stored by the computer, in spite of being repeatedly encouraged to do so. These results replicate earlier findings [Siegler and Liebert, 1975] that uninstructed preadolescents almost never spontaneously used records for planning factorial experiments, in spite of a strong correlation between keeping records and producing the full set of combinations of variables relevant in an experimental design task. Four children recorded nothing at all. The remaining 14 children recorded information that was uninformative. (For example, one child carefully recorded the outcome speed of every car without including any information about the features.)

Given these strategic weaknesses, how did children progress? First, recall that only 2 of the 22 children were able to correctly identify all the causal relations after 7 sessions. Over half the children failed even to identify all the simple causal relations. Specifically, children often maintained or reverted to earlier incorrect theories, using invalid data to support their interpretations. Those children whose strategies were especially weak had particular difficulties in changing their conviction that the muffler was causal, confirming earlier findings that it is easier to learn that a variable believed noncausal is in fact causal, than it is to learn that a variable believed causal is in fact noncausal [Kuhn et al., 1988]. Second, the progress, although real, was slow. By comparison, an adult scientist who performed the task successfully completed it in a single session containing 7 experiments, systematically testing each feature in turn and then searching for possible interactions. In contrast, children often generated the same cars over and over, changed their judgments about a feature an average of 20 times over the sessions, and failed finally to come to either a definitive or entirely correct solution. Nonetheless, all children showed some appropriate belief change and almost half discovered all effects except the interaction.

Often children appeared to be relying on a broad inductive method, that is, noting over a large number of cases that in general a variable level (e.g., a large engine) was or was not associated with faster cars. Many of them employed certain cars, whose outcomes they recalled, as prototypes.

For example, a child might recall the speed of a particular car that was the 'fastest car' or a 'car like my uncle's' or a 'little slow one with nothing on it.' Children then used these cars as a benchmark for comparison, generating predictions about the speed of novel cars on the basis of their similarity to the prototypes. As implied by contemporary theories of induction [e.g., Holland et al., 1986], given enough cases, these methods often lead to correct belief revision. However, as is also suggested by models like that proposed by Holland et al., when prior beliefs are not correct, they are unlikely to be rejected on the first encounter with disconfirming evidence, or in some cases, on several encounters. And although current analyses of scientific discovery [e.g., Klahr and Dunbar, 1988] indicate that good discoverers are strongly driven by theory, our children's performance illustrates that this characteristic may be problematic when theories are not correct. When they are not right, and failing any system of checks in which events take on evidential status in relation to beliefs, one finds a process perhaps better described as an unconscious drift over time toward a more correct understanding, rather than a process of reasoned theory revision. Supporting this characterization is the fact that much of the time, children seemed entirely unaware that they had changed a belief, even after having done so several times in close succession.

College Adults' Exploration of the Race Cars Microworld

We can now ask how characteristic of preadolescent children the preceding behavior is. Would a group of adults proceed in a qualitatively different way? This question is addressed by reviewing data from another study in which a group of undergraduates were introduced to an abbreviated version of the race cars microworld.

Twelve undergraduates participated in the study, 4 men and 8 women. Subjects were recruited and paid $5.00 per hour for participating. Participants worked at an initial session with the race cars microworld and then at subsequent sessions with a series of other scientific discovery tasks. The adults, unlike the children, were permitted to terminate their experimentation 'as soon as you are sure you have figured out what makes a difference and what does not make a difference in how fast a car can drive.'

The adults proceeded somewhat faster than the children did but on average made slightly less overall progress, largely because they terminated their experimentation prematurely (all within 30 min, and one person within 5 min). At the point when they announced that they understood the way the microworld worked, none of them had in fact discovered all the causal and noncausal relations (compared to 2 of the children) and only 4 of 12 were able to identify all relations except for the interaction (compared to 10 of the 22 children after seven weeks). The mean number of experiments that the adults conducted was only 5.0 (range 1–11), and the mean number of cars constructed was only 11.4 (range 2–21). A rough comparison is provided by the data from the children's first weekly session. During this first session, the children produced less information than the adults did; their mean number of experiments was 3.8 (range 3–8), and the mean number of cars constructed was 8.7 (range 7–12).

Both adults and children were influenced by belief, but the adults were somewhat less influenced than the children. Like the children's, the adults' theories about the muffler and tailfin were often initially wrong and thus could be disconfirmed by the microworld, in contrast to their theories about the engine and color. At the end of the session, the adults, like the children, better understood the effects of features that were consistent with their prior beliefs than those that were inconsistent. In fact, all 12 adults identified the simple-effects features that confirmed their initial beliefs, the engine and color. However, after completing their experiments, 3 of the 12 retained their initial incorrect beliefs about the muffler, and 2 retained their initial incorrect beliefs about the tailfin. By comparison, after 7 weeks, all of the children except one had achieved a correct understanding of the engine and color, comparable to the achievement of the adults. Also comparable to the adults, 5 of the 22 children persisted in judging that the muffler was causal. In contrast to the adults, however, 7 of 22 either judged the fin noncausal or incorrectly stated that cars with tailfins were faster than those without. Thus, both adults and children were influenced by prior beliefs, but even after 7 sessions, children on average did not achieve as much belief change as adults achieved in a single session. Overall, however, the pattern of adults' belief change looks remarkably like that of the children, although adults proceeded more quickly.

Generation of Evidence

When we examine the experimentation strategies that the adults employed, however, it becomes clear that, unlike children's, adults' activity more closely approximated a normative scientific reasoning cycle that includes strategies for designing and interpreting experiments. First, the adults did not repeatedly change their judgments concerning the causal status of design features. Unlike the children, they typically performed one experiment to learn about each feature, made a judgment on the basis of that experiment, and then went on to the next feature, until they had reached a conclusion about each in turn. When this point was reached, they announced that they were finished (although in some cases an adult simply forgot that he or she had neglected to test one or more features). Second, in contrast to children, adults were far more likely to vary only one variable at a time, and to make conclusions based on experiments that were, for the most part, valid.

Interpretation of Evidence

Because the children did not hesitate to draw definitive conclusions based on their imperfect experiments, many of their conclusions were incorrect, especially those that supported their prior beliefs about features. When the analysis is restricted only to data from the children's first session, we find that only a small percentage – a mean of 12% – of the children's judgments were valid (that is, judgments that were both correct and based on adequate evidence). In contrast, a mean of 68% of the adults' judgments were valid, although there was considerable variability even among these 12 adults (percentage of judgments that were valid ranged from 0% for one subject to 100% for 3 others). Further indication that the adults were attending more closely to the evidence comes from the fact that of the adults' judgments, very few were justified by reference to a prior belief about cars or mechanisms. Five adults each made one belief-based judgment, and only one adult made judgments that were predominantly based on theory. (This adult conducted only one experiment before announcing that she understood the microworld and then reported a series of judgments all based on her prior theories.) The adults tended to justify their judgments by referring directly to evidence from the experiments. Fewer than one-tenth of their judgments were initially justified by reference to theory or beliefs, in contrast to one-quarter of the children's. A final important difference lies in the kinds of inferences adults and children made. The clearest difference between the children's and adults' inference is in the adults' ability to make valid judgments of exclusion, i.e., judgments that a variable does not covary with outcome and thus does not play a causal role. Adults' valid judgments were about equally divided between inferences of inclusion and exclusion. In contrast, children made very few valid exclusion judgments. Adults rarely made invalid exclusion judgments, but children did so relatively frequently. These findings are consistent with previous research reporting that the inference strategy of valid exclusion is especially difficult for children to master [Kuhn et al., 1988].

Data Management

With respect to record-keeping, once again the performance of the adults was variable but was notably better than the children's. Recall that none of the children systematically recorded all information concerning both variables and outcomes in their logbooks. In contrast, half of the adults' notes were complete or nearly complete records of the covariation among variables and outcomes.

The preceding comparisons are of course not definitive; adults worked for only one session, and children worked for 7. In addition, adults were free to terminate whenever they wished to do so. Nevertheless, differences are apparent in the performances of children and college adults, suggesting the superiority of adults in several important dimensions of scientific reasoning, including design of controlled experiments, control of belief intrusion, mastery of exclusion inference, and metacognitive skills of data management.

However, the appropriateness of comparing adults and children working on the race cars task can be debated. Although the content and complexity of the race cars task was designed to be moderately challenging for 10-year-olds, it is certainly conceivable that the performance of college adults may have been affected by the fact that they were working on a problem that they did not perceive as challenging. Given an experimentation context that was for them comparably complex, the performance of college adults might appear more like that of children. This issue is now addressed by examining the performance of 30 undergraduate students working with the computer laboratory in economics.

Undergraduates' Exploration of a Microeconomics Laboratory

In Smithtown [Shute, Glaser, and Raghavan, 1989] undergraduate students first choose a market to explore (markets are goods or services for production and sale, such as coffee, typewriters, gasoline, and water). They then make changes in one or more independent variables (for example, the price of the good, the population of the town, or the number of suppliers), and, if desired, make one or more predictions about the outcomes of their manipulations. The computer then displays the effect of these changes on a number of related dependent variables (such as quantity supplied, quantity demanded, and surplus). The student has the option of permanently recording as much of this information as desired into an online notebook. He or she may also use a spreadsheet-like table package to sort the data in various ways or a graphing tool to graph relations in the data. Finally, the student uses a hypothesis menu to state the laws or principles that he or she is discovering; the computer evaluates the hypothesis for accuracy and indicates whether the student has generated sufficient data to support the conclusion.

Generation of Evidence

A number of activities differentiated successful from unsuccessful students, (i.e., those who made large vs. small or negligible gains in understanding). First, in the category of evidence generation, our better subjects were more likely to generate and test experimental predictions, i.e., their experiments were more likely to be hypothesis-driven. In contrast, less successful subjects tended to be data-driven. They manipulated variables and generated data without being guided by an experimental question of interest or an expectation about the probable outcome. As a consequence, the data they produced were not brought to bear on a developing understanding of the way Smithtown worked or put to use to confirm or disconfirm hypotheses. Recall the tendency of children to repeatedly change their judgments about variables in the race cars microworld. They appeared to be treating experiments as unrelated cases, rather than trying to develop a consistent and cumulative understanding of the effects of all the variables operating together. Like these children, the less successful undergraduates working in Smithtown appeared not to be using hypotheses to guide their experimentation or using their results to revise their hypotheses.

The better learners in Smithtown explored each economic market in greater depth, following through on an issue or an idea rather than jumping from market to market. They were also more likely than the poor learners to use effective experimental heuristics, such as carrying out experiments that varied only one variable at a time, holding all other variables constant. In contrast, the poorer subjects often changed several variables and then were unable to draw a definitive conclusion about the variable responsible for an outcome. Their behavior parallels that of the children who failed to design valid experiments in their work with the race cars microworld. As reported, children were much less likely than college adults to design informative and valid experiments with the race cars. The results from the Smithtown study show that when adults have difficulties with a more complex task, the generation of experiments is likely to be a source of difficulty for college undergraduates, as well.

Interpretation of Evidence

In interpreting evidence, the better Smithtown students were more likely to try to generalize a newly-discovered economic concept to different markets or contexts, to see how widely it applied. In contrast, less successful subjects rarely checked a relation to see if it held in new cases. Once again, there are parallels to subjects' behavior in Daytona, the race cars world. However, recall that with the race cars, both adults and children drew conclusions based on insufficient data. The adults, like the children, were quick to jump to conclusions, almost never checking, for example, to see whether a relation held consistently when other features on a car were varied. As a consequence, very few subjects (either adults or children) noted the interaction between engine and tailfin. In the Smithtown study, the better students frequently manipulated an independent variable several times, and then observed the outcome to make sure the result was consistent. In contrast, less successful subjects often made careless or impulsive generalizations based on inadequate data. To some extent, this behavior parallels that of children in the Daytona study who observed a fast car with a muffler and then claimed this outcome as 'proof' that a fast car must have a muffler. In Daytona, such misunderstanding of the nature of covariation evidence was most characteristic of children; only one adult subject misinterpreted data in this way. However, in Smithtown, drawing conclusions on the basis of insufficient evidence was a common pitfall for the poorer subjects.

Data Management

In the third category of interest, recording and managing data, parallels in the Smithtown and Daytona results also appear. The better Smithtown students were more likely than poorer ones to systematically record data from their experiments in their on-line notebook and were also more likely to record relevant data, i.e., data regarding the variables they were currently exploring. In Daytona, recall, very few children used their logbooks in an informative way, whereas more (but by no means all) of the adults did so.

Conclusions: Age Differences in Scientific Thinking

In summary, when both children and college adults worked on the same task (a task designed to be challenging to preadolescents), differences occurred in how they went about solving the problem. However, a comparable group of adults working on a more complex discovery problem looked more like the children in the first task. Dunbar and Klahr [1989] have also compared the performance of college adults and children working on a discovery task, and they found that children, in contrast to adults, showed errors like those reported here: generating uninformative experiments, jumping to conclusions on the basis of minimal and inconclusive evidence, and making inconsistent and vacillating judgments. However, if such differences can be erased by changing the task complexity, in what sense do strategies in scientific experimentation develop?

Certainly the variability in the performance of our subjects indicates that it is not the case that all children lack these skills and all adults possess them. Even when individuals from different age groups participate in the same task, variability in performance within an age group is the rule, not the exception. Clearly these findings are not consonant with simple structuralist models of development, nor are they consistent with any theory of reasoning that regards strategies as being applied in a generalized manner independent of context or content. Our research suggests that variables that affect reasoning include (but are not limited to) subjects' familiarity or practice with the activity, content knowledge about the domain, and the demands of the task. Contemporary developmental theorists [Fischer, 1980; Fischer and Farrar, 1988; Siegler and Jenkins, 1989] concentrate on articulating mechanisms of development that can account for these influences, including specifying possible relations between developmental change that is characterized by gradual, incremental acquisition, and comprehensive, qualitative changes in related complexes of behaviors.

Given objectively similar tasks, children typically fail to use strategies that most adults apparently use spontaneously. However, these strategies are not perfectly mastered by adults; they are not always employed where they would be useful, and their use can be disrupted by increasing the complexity of the task or the task's dependence on domain knowledge, or both. In these cases, both adults and children may fail to attend to evidence. Adults as well as children often fail to control for extraneous variation in their experiments and make invalid conclusions based on confounded or insufficient evidence. As a consequence, they frequently judge that variables are causal when they cannot definitively identify the effect of that variable in isolation and have particular difficulties correctly interpreting evidence that there is no causal relation between a variable and an outcome.

Given this pattern of results, the most profitable way of posing the developmental question is to ask how strategies in scientific experimentation change over time and what supports that change. The kinds of skills described here are rarely the focus of direct instruction; even instruction in elementary school often assumes that they are already in place. While our data and the studies of others [Dunbar and Klahr, 1989] indicate that most adults typically outperform most children, equally convincing is the evidence that when children are given concentrated practice in the use of these skills, they show steady improvement over a short period of time [Kuhn and Phelps, 1982; Schauble, 1990].

A few explanations for these changes have been proposed. One proposal is that with time and practice, an individual's metacognitive awareness of a particular strategy improves; that is, one becomes more aware of the advantages and disadvantages of using one strategy as opposed to another. Kuhn [1989] points out that it is not only acquiring new, more effective strategies that subjects find problematic, but rather giving up earlier-mastered, less effective ones. She suggests that over time, subjects are coming to understand the advantages of the newer strategies, so that they can deploy them reflectively in an appropriate way.

However, Siegler and Jenkins [1989] point out that there is another explanation consistent with the finding that subjects fail to suddenly abandon their older, less effective strategies when they generate newer, more appropriate ones. Their explanation is that strategies are stored in memory as rules, each candidate rule associated with a strength value that derives from its previous usefulness in predicting real-world outcomes. Strategies or rules compete with one another, in the sense that several may be simultaneously present and active, yet in any given situation the strategy that is selected for use will be the rule with the greatest strength at the time of selection. The implication is that a person need not be consciously aware of or reflective about a strategy before it begins to play a more important role in the overall repertoire of behaviors. However, Siegler and Jenkins suggest that there may be a connection between being conscious of using a strategy and the full and consistent use of that strategy.

A third possibility, one that we have recently begun to explore, is that individuals differently understand the objective of scientific experimentation, and that the way they construe the goal affects the kinds of strategies employed. The process of experimentation involves generating, executing, and coordinating a number of subgoals, such as developing one or more hypotheses, designing an experiment to test a hypothesis, making a prediction about the outcome, observing and interpreting the result, and recording data. Not only do subjects vary with respect to their ability to carry out parts of the process, but they also appear to vary with respect to their understanding of the goal and subgoals involved, including why they are engaging in these activities, and the relation of the various components to each other. For example, children working with the race cars often proceeded as if constructing cars and making predictions about their speeds was an activity entirely unrelated to observing the cars and interpreting the outcome. Thus, a child might design a car and predict a speed, e.g., 'This car will go to flag 3'. Upon observing that the car in fact only went to flag 1, it was not atypical for a child to construct the same car again and to make the same prediction about its speed.

Other researchers report observations consistent with the interpretation that children are not sure what they are supposed to be doing when they are asked to engage in experimentation. One solution they may invent is to substitute a more familiar, alternative goal. Typically, they try to reproduce a favored or interesting outcome. For example, when Tschirgi [1980] asked children to indicate which of several experiments would be optimal for determining what ingredients would produce a cake that turned out either 'terrible' or 'great', she found that children selected experiments that reproduced the conditions resulting in good cakes. Kuhn and Phelps [1982] studied the experimental strategies that children deployed in trying to determine which chemical in a mixture was responsible for a reaction in which the mixture turned pink. They found that instead of trying to determine the causes of the chemical reaction, some children persisted in designing experiments that would replicate it. In the race cars study, children were frequently distracted from the stated goal of the task (find out what makes a difference in the speed of a car) by an attractive alternative goal that they spontaneously generated – trying to build the fastest possible car. The effect of this reinterpretation of the goal was that a child trying to produce fast cars could achieve this objective without attending at all to the role of the features that were *not* causal. These children often failed to realize that certain features were playing no causal role and thus could be eliminated from further consideration. In addition, if one's goal is to make fast cars (or a great cake, or a pink mixture), setting up valid experiments that isolate variables is not the fastest way to proceed. Instead, it may be more efficient to engage in a 'focus gambling' strategy [Bruner et al., 1956] – that is, constructing a car that includes *all* variables suspected to make the car faster. If the car does not turn out to be the fastest, one then changes each manipulable feature in turn until the desired outcome is obtained. In this sense, the interpretation of the task objective can drive strategy selection.

It is not only children who form their own interpretations of the goal of scientific inquiry. In the work with Smithtown, some of our undergraduates developed an alternative interpretation of their objective that is similar to those that the children developed with the race cars. Instead of trying to discern relations in the data so that they could determine causes and effects, some students acted as if they believed their task was to make certain kinds of outcomes occur – for example, to achieve equilibrium in a particular market or to produce financial success for the inhabitants of Smithtown.

Results relevant to this issue have been obtained from a study of 23 undergraduate nonscience majors who worked for an extended period of time with our computer-based circuit laboratory, Voltaville. Before each experiment, an interviewer asked, 'What are you going to learn with this experiment?' or 'What are you trying to accomplish here?' Students' responses to these queries were coded as their goals or plans for the experiment that immediately followed. Differences in students' plans reflected fundamentally different understandings of the experimentation task they were engaged in. Those students who made little progress in discovering the principles of electricity tended to state plans that were local and task-oriented; they most often mentioned completing component parts of the task of operating the computer laboratory such as, 'I'm going to choose the next circuit in the menu,' or 'I guess I will measure voltage.' These students appeared to focus on completing each operational step in turn, losing sight of the overall goal of their activity and needing to be repeatedly reminded that the point was to identify the principles or laws. In contrast, more successful students stated plans concerning objectives like finding relations, generalizing relations to new cases, or resolving anomalies in the data they were observing, for example, 'I want to see if resistance works the same way in the parallel circuit as it did in the series circuit,' or, 'I want to figure out how the total resistance can be a smaller value than the resistance of one resistor.' Our surmise is that the poorer students either did not have a clear picture of the goal of experimentation or they had difficulties holding that goal in mind so that it effectively organized their activity.

Thus, the kind of search or reasoning that people employ will vary with their interpretation of the goal state. The implication is that in addition to concentrating on the scientific reasoning strategies that individuals do or do not display, it is important to attend to their interpretation of the task, and ask how that develops as well. Experimentation is an ill-formed problem that involves framing questions, planning a way to address them, and deciding when a conclusion is satisfactory. It is easy to see why relative novices, whether children or adults, find such a task ambiguous. The question we and others [e.g., Dunbar, 1989] are now beginning to attend to is how an individual comes to understand what experimentation is all about and how that understanding evolves. We believe that this kind of understanding serves to organize performance of the kinds of strategies we have described in our subjects' reasoning, including avoiding belief bias, developing controlled experiments, making valid interpretations of data, taking account of experimental evidence, and engaging in reasoned belief revision.

Implications for Education

These findings suggest that research can contribute to the knowledge teachers require to assist students in developing a more stable, elaborated, and rich understanding of scientific inquiry. The typical introductory text chapter describing the scientific method is inadequate to this end. Rather than imparting a set of principles that can be memorized and acquired once and for all, we need to search for effective ways of supporting a kind of understanding that continues to evolve over an extended period of time. We suggest that such an understanding encompasses intimate connections between domain knowledge and conceptions, purposes and goals of a problem situation, and strategies of experimentation of the kind that we have been describing here.

Instruction needs to focus on the enablement offered by both domain knowledge and the thinking skills fundamental to science. Glaser [1984] and Resnick [1987] have suggested that the most effective way of bringing reasoning into school instruction may not be presenting specialized courses or curriculum devoted to thinking skills or higher-order reasoning, but by incorporating reasoning and problem solving into the acquisition of knowledge in school subjects. It is not enough for our students to simply learn facts and concepts; in addition, we must help them learn how to reason with that knowledge. Learning to reason in science domains, we suggest, is fundamentally different both from learning general principles or heuristics of reasoning and from learning about science content. When specific knowledge domains are taught in interactive, interrogative ways, students exercise general thinking skills and the inferential power of their growing domain knowledge. The ability to use a rich network of domain concepts and a repertoire of flexible and productive experimental and inferential strategies is fundamental to competence in scientific inquiry.

Acknowledgements

Preparation of this chapter was sponsored in part by the Center for the Study of Learning (CSL) at the Learning Research and Development Center of the University of Pittsburgh. CSL is funded by the Office of Educational Research and Improvement of the U.S. Department of Education. *Smithtown, Voltaville,* and *Refract* were developed in collaboration with Kalyani Raghavan, Jamie Schultz, Mayura Channarasappa, Valerie Shute, and Peter Reimann. *Daytona* was developed in collaboration with Jonathan Cohen, Deanna Kuhn, and Angela Greene.

References

Brown, A.L., & DeLoache, J.S. (1978). Skills, plans, and self-regulation. In R.S. Siegler (Ed.), *Children's thinking: What develops?* (pp. 3–36). Hillsdale NJ: Erlbaum.

Bruner, J.W., Goodnow, J.J., & Austin, G.A. (1956). *A study of thinking.* New York: New York Sciences Editions, Inc.

Chipman, S.F., Segal, J.W., & Glaser, R. (Eds.). (1985). *Thinking and learning Skills: Vol. 2. Research and open questions.* Hillsdale NJ: Erlbaum.

Dunbar, K. (1989). Scientific reasoning strategies in a simulated molecular genetics environment. Paper presented at the annual meeting of the Cognitive Science Society, East Lansing, MI.

Dunbar. K., & Klahr, D. (1989). Development differences in scientific discovery strategies. In D. Klahr & K. Kotovsky (Eds.), *Complex information processing: The impact of Herbert A. Simon* (pp. 109–144). Hillsdale NJ: Erlbaum.

Einhorn H.J., & Hogarth, R.M. (1986). Judging probable cause. *Psychological Bulletin, 99,* 3–19.

Halpern, D.F. (1984). *Thought and knowledge: An introduction to critical thinking.* Hillsdale NJ: Erlbaum.

Fischer, K.W. (1980). A theory of cognitive development: The control and construction of hierarchies of skills. *Psychological Review, 87,* 477–531.

Fischer, K., & Farrar, M. (1988). Generalizations about generalization: How a theory of skill development explains both generality and specificity. In A. Demetriou (Ed.), *The neo-Piagetian theories of cognitive development: Toward an integration.* Amsterdam: Elsevier.

Glaser, R. (1984). Education and thinking: The role of knowledge. *American Psychologist, 39,* 93–104.

Glaser, R., Raghavan, K., & Schauble, L. (1988). Voltaville, a discovery environment to explore the laws of DC circuits. In *ITS-88* (Proceedings of the 1988 Intelligent Tutoring Systems Conference). Montreal, Quebec.

Holland, J.H., Holyoak, K.J., Nisbett, R.E., & Thagard, P.R. (1986). *Induction: Processes of inference, learning, and discovery.* Cambridge MA: MIT Press.

Karmiloff-Smith, A., & Inhelder, B. (1974). If you want to get ahead, get a theory. *Cognition, 3,* 195–212.

Klahr, D., & Dunbar, K. (1988). Dual search space during scientific reasoning. *Cognitive Science, 12,* 1–48.

Klayman, J., & Ha, Y. (1987). Confirmation, disconfirmation and information in hypothesis testing. *Psychological Review, 94,* 211–228.

Kuhn, D. (1989). Children and adults as intuitive scientists. *Psychological Review, 96,* 674–689.

Kuhn, D., Amsel, E., & O'Loughlin, M. (1988). *The development of scientific thinking skills.* Orlando FL: Academic Press.

Kuhn, D., & Phelps, E. (1982). The development of problem-solving strategies. In H.W. Reese (Ed.), *Advances in child development and behavior: Vol 17* (pp. 1–44). New York: Academic Press.

Mynatt, C.R., Doherty, M.E., & Tweney, R.D. (1977). Confirmation bias in a simulated research environment: An experimental study of scientific inference. *Quarterly Journal of Experimental Psychology, 29,* 85–95.

Nickerson, R.S., Perkins, D., & Smith, E.E. (1985). *The teaching of thinking.* Hillsdale NJ: Erlbaum.

Resnick, L.B. (1987). *Education and learning to think.* Washington DC: National Academy Press.

Robinson, L.B., & Hastie, R. (1985). Revision of beliefs when a hypothesis is eliminated from consideration. *Journal of Experimental Psychology: Human Perception and Performance, 11,* 443–456.

Schauble, L. (1990). Belief revision in children: The role of prior knowledge and strategies for generating evidence. *Journal of Experimental Child Psychology, 49,* 31–57.

Segal, J.W., Chipman, S.F., & Glaser, R., Eds. (1985). *Thinking and learning skills: Vol. 1. Relating instruction to research.* Hillsdale NJ: Erlbaum.

Shute, V., Glaser, R., & Raghavan, K. (1989). Inference and discovery in an exploratory laboratory. In P.L. Ackerman, R.J. Sternberg, & R. Glaser (Eds.), *Learning and individual differences: Advances in theory and research* (pp. 279–326). New York: Freeman.

Siegler, R.S., & Jenkins, R. (1989). *How children discover new strategies.* Hillsdale NJ: Erlbaum.

Siegler, R.S., & Liebert, R.M. (1975). Acquisition of formal scientific reasoning by 10- and 13-year-olds: Designing a factorial experiment. *Developmental Psychology, 11,* 401–402.

Simon, H.A., & Kotovsky, K. (1963). Human acquisition of concepts for sequential patterns. *Psychological Review, 70,* 534–546.

Tschirgi, J.E. (1980). Sensible reasoning: A hypothesis about hypotheses. *Child Development, 51,* 1–10.

Wason, P.C. (1968). Reasoning about a rule. *Quarterly Journal of Experimental Psychology, 20,* 273–281.

Kuhn D (ed): Developmental Perspectives on Teaching and Learning Thinking Skills.
Contrib Hum Dev. Basel, Karger, 1990, vol 21, pp 28–47

Harmful Heuristics and the Improvement of Thinking

Jonathan Baron

One approach to thinking instruction emphasizes what I have called actively open-minded thinking [Baron, 1988a, 1989]. Students are taught to consider alternative possibilities, neglected goals, and counterevidence. The basic psychological claim is that people are overconfident – in their beliefs, decisions, and choices of goals – because they have been biased toward views they favor initially. The claim is not that people ought to be actively open-minded about everything but rather that they should not be confident in their conclusions unless they have reached them with this kind of scrutiny. Similar views have been put forward by Nickerson [1989], Paul [1984], Perkins [in press], and Perkins et al. [1986].

Another approach to thinking instruction emphasizes heuristics, that is, general rules of search or inference that people sometimes follow. Some, like Schoenfeld [1985], emphasize the positive value of heuristics in fields such as mathematics. Others, such as the contributors to the 1982 volume by Kahneman, Slovic, and Tversky, emphasize the need to overcome harmful heuristics in judgment and decision-making.

In this paper, I suggest that the absence of actively open-minded thinking, over the course of development, leads to the formation of harmful heuristics in judgments and decisions. In part, this is because harmful heuristics are overgeneralizations of helpful heuristics that are poorly understood by those who use them, and understanding, in turn, results from actively open-minded thinking. The implication of this argument, if it is true, is that when we teach heuristics we should try to induce students to understand why the helpful ones are helpful and why the harmful ones are harmful. When we try to induce such understanding, it should be through actively open-minded thinking.

Actively Open-Minded Thinking

The approach to thinking that I have taken begins with an analysis of real-life thinking tasks, including, but not limited to, those done in school [Baron, 1985, ch. 3]. Given a general description of thinking as it occurs in daily life, we can proceed to ask about the nature of good thinking and of the kinds of departures from this ideal that occur. The answers to these questions, in turn, will provide us with a standard by which to judge the effects of education and other sources of intellectual development. The advantages of this approach are that it reduces the probability of fixing things that are not broken and increases the probability of helping children, and the adults they become, to cope with tasks beyond those that we invent.

Thinking is a conscious response to doubt. It is what we do when we are at a loss, at least for a moment, about what to do or what to believe. For example, some of my stock has declined in value recently. What should I do?

We may analyze all thinking into search and inference. We search for possibilities, evidence, and goals. Possibilities are possible answers to my question: do nothing; sell the stock and buy other stock; sell it and buy bonds; buy more of it. I may think of possibilities myself, or people may suggest them to me. Evidence is anything I use to decide among the possibilities, such as reports about the economy and general principles of investing. Goals are the criteria I use to weigh the evidence. How much do I care about safety versus growth? Goals are not all given. I have to search for them and sometimes discover what they are, just as I search for evidence. I might discover the goal of investing as a way of expressing my politics, or the goal of avoiding worry. The *use of evidence*, in light of goals, to strengthen or weaken possibilities, is inference. Inference relies on heuristics and other kinds of rules. Inference is only part of thinking, however; the rest is search.

Thinking goes wrong in two ways. First, our search misses something that it should have discovered. For example, I may neglect to consider evidence about the uncertainty of future bond prices resulting from interest-rate changes. I may fail to consider possibilities such as paying off part of my mortgage. I may neglect goals such as liquidity when I need the money for a child's education. Neglect of goals often results from single-mindedness, e.g., pursuing the goal of minimizing risk above all else.

The second way in which thinking goes wrong is that we make incorrect inferences from the evidence we have, often because we use faulty heuristics. For example, I could decide against selling the stock because selling at a loss would be a waste of the money that I invested. I might be using a heuristic that tells me not to take any action that results in an uncompensated loss. This heuristic is applicable only when I have a choice in advance. The heuristic tells me not to decide to throw money away without a return. The purpose of this heuristic is to alert us to possible losses and make us search for less wasteful alternatives. If I thought about the rule against waste in an actively open-minded way, searching for goals and for alternative rules, I would possibly discover that the heuristic does not serve its goal when the loss has already occurred. I would then consider an alternative heuristic, which tells me not to choose options that result in future uncompensated loss.

Very often, poor thinking involves ignoring evidence against a possibility that the thinker initially favors. The same favoritism may cause us to cut off prematurely our search for alternatives to our initial idea or for reasons why it might be wrong. By contrast, good thinking consists of search that is thorough in proportion to the importance of the question, and includes fairness to other possibilities than the one we initially favor. It is such thinking that I earlier referred to as 'actively open-minded'. Confidence in the results of thinking is unwarranted unless the thinking has been actively open-minded. If we do not seek reasons why we are wrong, we can miss them.

Of course, we may think too much, or we may be too self-critical. I have argued [Baron, 1985, 1988a], however, that these errors are the less common ones. Actively open-minded thinking is a virtue, like thrift, that should be practiced in moderation, and with sensitivity to the demands of the situation, but it is still a virtue. We consider thrift a virtue because most people are not thrifty enough, even though some people are misers.

Actively open-minded thinking, when induced in the laboratory, can reduce overconfidence and self-serving biases [Koriat et al., 1980; Hoch, 1985]. Some findings can be interpreted as showing large effects of education level [Kuhn, forthcoming], although other studies show only small effects [Perkins, 1985]. Actively open-minded thinking can clearly be improved by special courses designed to teach it [Perkins, in press; Perkins et al., 1986]. To some extent, actively open-minded thinking seems to be a disposition that results from the thinker's own standards. Those who engage in it believe that this is the way that people should think. Those who do not tend to think that it is more important to be loyal to one's initial view [Baron, 1989; in press]. Education in actively open-minded thinking can therefore go a long way by changing students' beliefs about what good thinking is.

Heuristics and Biases

In recent years, evidence has accumulated showing that people are subject to systematic biases in judgment and decision-making [Arkes and Hammond, 1986; Baron, 1985, 1988a [part III]; Kahneman et al., 1982; Kahneman and Tversky, 1984; Thaler, 1985]. Consider the following: (1) People who will not pay as much as $X for a coupon will not sell the same coupon for more than $X [Knetsch and Sinden, 1984], even though both decisions could be described as a choice between $X and the coupon. (2) Judgments of decision quality are influenced by outcomes that the decision-maker could not have foreseen [Baron and Hershey, 1988]. (3) Costs already 'sunk' into a project lead people to continue the project even though they would not continue on the basis of future costs and benefits alone [Arkes and Blumer, 1985]. The list of such biases is long.

Most of these biases violate certain principles of rational choice, as embodied in the various forms of utility theory. According to utility theory, the best option maximizes utility, which may be defined [Baron, 1988a] as a measure of the extent to which the outcomes of the choice achieve the decision maker's goals. Uncertainty about outcomes is taken into account by multiplying the utility of each outcome by its probability. When people violate utility theory, they subvert their own goals [Baron, 1988a, part III; Baron, in preparation].

Biases that violate utility theory can usually be ascribed to the use of decision heuristics, or rules of thumb. Some heuristics are easily seen as erroneous by those who use them, but, at the other end of a continuum, other heuristics are deeply held and do not yield easily to arguments. An example of the latter is some people's belief in basing decisions on 'worst-case scenarios,' rather than on their best judgments of probabilities, when they feel that their probability judgments could be greatly affected by information they lack [Frisch and Baron, 1988]. The fact that people resist changing their heuristics does not mean that their heuristics are correct. What makes a heuristic best is not whether users accept it but whether it best serves their goals.

The use of heuristics that lead to bias is not necessarily irrational, for decision-makers in the real world rarely have the time or ability even to approximate the calculations required to make the best possible decision. We are often forced to rely on our intuitions. A distinction thus emerges between normative and prescriptive theories of rationality [Baron, 1985, 1986, 1988a, 1988b]. A normative theory, such as utility theory, provides an ultimate standard of rational decision-making. A prescriptive theory of rationality recognizes human limitations and tells us how we can go about making the best decisions in practice. A good prescriptive theory should be sensitive to the demands of limited time and other constraints, yet should yield a pattern of decisions that approximates what would have been obtained with the normative theory itself. A good normative theory should provide a standard for discussing how well prescriptive methods achieve the goals we have for them. Although the normative-prescriptive distinction implies that heuristics that fall short of the normative ideal are not necessarily irrational, it does not imply that they are rational in the sense of being the best we could achieve. We could discover other heuristics whose benefit in better meeting the normative standard is greater than their cost (if any) in difficulty of learning them.

We can find biases in decisions that affect others, as well as those that affect only the self. For example, Spranca et al. [in press] have found that many subjects make an unjustified distinction between omission and commission in deciding what to do or in judging the decisions of others. In one study, subjects were asked to evaluate medical policies for treating a serious disease. In one condition, 20% of the patients would be brain-damaged by the disease; the treatment (which completely cured the disease) would cause the same damage in 15%. In another condition, the probabilities were reversed. Across both conditions, subjects rated omission (no treatment) as a better policy. A small but significant number of subjects even rated no treatment as better than treatment in the first condition, when more people would suffer brain damage with this 'better' no-treatment policy. Ritov and Baron [1989] similarly found that many subjects prefer not to vaccinate children when the vaccine can kill the children, even though the death rate from the vaccination is a mere fraction of the death rate from the disease it prevents.

Where Do Harmful Heuristics Come from?

Let us assume that a decision or judgment is examined as a function of various factors (some of which are the results of other judgments). For example, judgments of an actor's morality could be affected by such factors as the actor's judged motives and intentions, the goodness or badness of the consequences the actor caused, whether the consequences resulted from the actor's omission or commission, whether they were foreseeable, whether people think an action is bad, whether an actor's role requirements have been violated, and so on. A judge will attend to certain factors and ignore others.

For any decision or judgment, a normative theory will specify what factors should influence the decision. The standard here is that factors are relevant when attending to them helps us achieve our goals. 'Our' here is intentionally ambiguous. For purely personal decisions, the goals are those of the decision-maker. For decisions that affect other people and that we evaluate from an impersonal, moral perspective, 'our' goals are everyone's goals.

Biases result when factors are misweighed relative to one another, when relevant factors are ignored, or when irrelevant factors are used in making a judgment or decision. I shall ignore misweighing here and focus on the two latter types of bias.

Attending to Irrelevant Factors

Attention to irrelevant factors rarely appears to be totally unreasonable. Why is this?

Contingent Relevance and Overgeneralization

Some factors are normatively relevant sometimes but not at other times, depending on the availability of information about other factors. These factors are contingently relevant. They are relevant only in case certain other information, with which they are correlated, is not available. If we are hiring an assistant professor, an applicant's Graduate Record Examination scores would be relevant information if (implausibly) we knew nothing about her performance in graduate school. The relevance of the test, however, disappears when the information about graduate school performance is available. The GRE score is contingently relevant. Most of the known biases that involve use of irrelevant factors concern contingently relevant factors. This is so, I propose, because biases often result from overgeneralization of heuristics from cases in which they are relevant to those in which they are not. Because the factors are sometimes relevant, attention to them does not seem totally unreasonable.

Overgeneralization occurs because people do not understand the purposes of the heuristics they use, that is, the relation of the heuristics to the normative models that justify them or to the idea of optimal goal achievement. If people come to understand that certain heuristics are useful because they help to maximize utility or bring our judgments closer to the truth, then people can learn to recognize when these conditions are not met. For example, people tend to judge the quality of others' decisions according to the outcome of the decision, like 'Monday-morning quarterbacks.' But outcome information is useful for such judgment only because it is correlated with relevant information available to the decision-maker but not to the judge. When all relevant information is available to the judge, outcome is irrelevant. People persist in using it anyway [Baron and Hershey, 1988; Spranca et al., in press], but that is perhaps because they fail to understand why it is useful.

Understanding

Students and their teachers often make a distinction between understanding something and 'just memorizing' it (or perhaps not learning it at all). Learning of heuristics can occur in either of these ways. I hypothesize that heuristics learned with understanding will transfer more appropriately and therefore will not be so frequently misapplied.

Wertheimer [1945/1959] and Katona [1940] argued that learning transfers appropriately to new cases only when understanding has occurred. For example, Wertheimer found that students who had learned the base-times-height formula for the area of the parallelogram would apply the same formula to other figures (such as trapezoids) that could not be made into rectangles in the way that parallelograms can be. Wertheimer (perhaps following Duncker, [1945]), suggested that understanding has something to do with knowledge of purpose. Perkins [1986] elaborates this kind of account of understanding: To understand, you must not only know the purpose of the 'structure' at issue but you must also know the arguments (evidence) about why that structure serves the purpose. For example, in the case of the parallelogram, one argument explaining why the formula gives the area is that the parallelogram has the same area as a rectangle of the same base and height.

This analysis of understanding explains the fact that principles that are understood do not transfer inappropriately. In solving the problems to which the base-times-height formula does not apply, the use of purpose as a retrieval cue may call forth the same knowledge as in solving the problems for which the formula is appropriate, but the search for arguments will not succeed. If the original arguments (about being able to make the figure into a rectangle) are found, they will not apply. (See Baron, [1988a], pp. 92–101, for additional discussion.)

In the case of heuristics, people learn without understanding because they do not think enough – or at all – about the heuristics that they use, and when they do think, they are not sufficiently actively open-minded. In particular, they do not search for goals (purposes) of these principles and for evidence (arguments) about why their rules serve their purposes in a given type of situation. In simple terms, people overgeneralize because they are unreflective. But I have tried to go beyond that label to indicate what kind of 'reflection' is missing.

Alternative Accounts

My proposal can be made clearer by contrasting it with two alternative accounts of the use of irrelevant factors. By one account, people may fail to learn from experience which heuristics are best because they make errors in testing and evaluating hypotheses about their own heuristics. This account assumes that people could learn about heuristics from trial-and-error, rather than through understanding, if they went about it correctly. Although I do not deny that this process occurs, I suspect that learning from experience (as opposed to learning by understanding or learning from others) does not occur as often as we often assume [see Brehmer, 1980]. Feedback is often not available, as in the making of moral judgments about others, the making of decisions that affect others but not oneself, or the making of decisions about one's own distant future.

Another possible account of apparent use of irrelevant factors is that the heuristics that people use *are* actually optimal when cognitive costs are considered. Payne et al. [1988; see also Christensen-Szalanski, 1978] have analyzed the use of heuristics in multi-attribute decisions in terms of such costs. They argue that lexicographic rules, in which a decision is made on the basis of a single factor, are less costly than compensatory rules, so lexicographic rules are used when time is short or when the decision is unimportant. If this account is sufficient, biases will not be reduced by understanding the purpose of heuristics or by learning from experience. Although this account may be true for some heuristics, it does not apply quite as easily to heuristics that involve attention to a factor that should be ignored, for this would seem to require more effort rather than less. (However, the effort could be in distinguishing those cases in which the factor is relevant from those in which it is not.) First-blush evidence against this view as sufficient is also provided by Nisbett et al. [1987], who found that education reduces certain biases in judgment, and by Larrick et al. [1989], who found that biases in economic decision-making are negatively correlated with economic success.

Neglect of Relevant Factors

People may neglect relevant factors because they elevate arguments into basic principles, or categorical rules, by which one consideration takes absolute priority over others. This happens often with arguments based on rights. We do not sell our right to free speech or our right to vote. Likewise, for some, the right to sue someone in court, to be compensated for harms caused by others, to drink clean water, and to trade in the marketplace assume privileged status.

Categorical rules have their advantages. When people try to trade off competing values or goals, they often err, either because of random error or self-serving bias. When the normative model would decide in favor of one consideration in the vast majority of cases, people can approximate the normative results better by following a categorical rule than by trying to make the optimal tradeoffs in each case. For example, although there are cases in which political terrorism is surely justified (e.g., to have stopped Hitler), the world would probably be a better place on the whole if it were never committed regardless of the apparent good that it could do.

Problems arise, however, when people elevate useful rules of thumb to the status of absolutes, without understanding that absolute rules can be justified only as means to a normative end, in the way just illustrated. Without such understanding, people take categorical intuitions to be their own justification, beyond criticism even when they conflict with other categorical intuitions. Doing so can lead to heated conflicts over many issues, such as national sovereignty, abortion, or the use of new medical procedures and biotechnologies. Conflicts between categorical rules can occur even within an individual. Concerning a case in which a boy died because his parents, Christian Scientists, refused medical treatment, Dershowitz [1988] commented, 'If ever there were a right that seemed absolute, it would be the right of the parents to bring up the child in their own religion. And if ever there were a right that seemed absolute, it would be the right of the child to receive adequate medical care. So here you have two absolute rights in direct conflict'. Categorical rules also lead to inconsistencies because we cannot consistently avoid the risk of violating them [Baron, 1986]. I may hold human life to be sacred, beyond any other consideration, but when I ask my mother to drive to the post office for me, I put her life on the line for the sake of a mere convenience.

The overuse of categorical rules can be explained in terms of a failure to search for goals and counterevidence. Categorical rules serve a single goal, but they typically conflict with achievement of other goals. People may persist in thinking that a categorical rule is good because they fail to consider the other goals when they think about the rule. They also fail to think of possible cases in which the rule does not work. As Hare [1981] pointed out, such examples do not prove that one should not follow the rule, as the terrorism example suggests. But they do give the rule a contingent status, requiring further justification in terms of ultimate ends.

Are categorical rules really held? Often, categorical rules are self-serving. When the tradeoff is risk against cost, for example, it is always those who do not have to pay the cost who argue that risk gets absolute priority, while those who do have to pay the cost speak of other rights such as economic freedom and the perfection of market forces. Categorical rules might be bargaining positions rather than psychological errors.

Laboratory evidence suggests that some categorical rules are truly held. Subjects have no reason to bargain with me when I ask them for their thoughts. If they behave as if they do, they have, for all practical purposes, adopted a rule as their own. In the vaccination study described earlier [Ritov and Baron, 1989], some subjects, when asked whether the government should require vaccinations even when the vaccinations could cause death, said that the government should not impose the vaccine unless it had zero risk of death. (Recall that the vaccine could lead to far less loss of life than the flu it prevented.) For example, one subject said, 'You can't force parents to give their kid a drug or vaccine that could cause the kid to die!'

I have found apparent use of such rules in other experiments in which subjects are asked to trade off one sort of consideration for another. For example, in another set of situations, I asked subjects how much of an increase in the cost of home heating oil should be tolerated as a cost of making antipollution regulations (for oil refineries) that would save lives (assuming various numbers of dollars per life saved). Fifteen of 53 subjects said that there was no limit on what should be spent, often justifying their answer with the assertion that human life was more important than money. (Of course, if subjects were consistent in their willingness to spend money to save lives, there are so many ways in which this could be done that money would be spent on nothing else.) Three other subjects said that no such government regulations should be allowed, apparently following exactly the opposite categorical rule.

Overgeneralization Error

In a number of biases, subjects use contingently relevant information even when they possess the necessarily relevant information with which it is correlated. These biases can be explained by assuming that subjects do not understand the rules heuristics for using the information. They do not relate these rules to their purposes.

Outcome Bias

The biases already mentioned are good examples. The outcome bias described by Baron and Hershey [1988] is one. Judgments of decisions were affected by the outcome of the decision, even when the judge was provided with all information the decision-maker had that was relevant. Spranca et al. [in press] found that a few subjects showed outcome bias even when the cases differing in outcome were presented one immediately following the other. The influence of outcome information, in this case, must be due to subjects' failure to recognize its lack of normative relevance. In other words, subjects lack understanding of the basis of their judgment. The outcome is useful in judgment when we do not know the outcomes and the probabilities available to the decision-maker. Other things equal, the outcome that occurred was more likely than other outcomes. But when we know the probabilities from the decision-maker's point of view, outcome is irrelevant. Here, the 'parallelogram' is the situation in which the judge does not know everything the decision-maker knew, and the 'trapezoid' – to which the rule is overgeneralized – is the situation in which the judge does know what the decision-maker knew.

Omission Bias

Another example of incorrect use of contingently relevant information, due to inadequate understanding of rules, is the use of information about whether an outcome was the result of an omission or a commission in judging the morality or prudence of a decision. Ordinarily, this variable is relevant because commissions are more strongly intended than omissions. But when subjects are fully informed about intention, some subjects still judge harmful omissions as worse [Spranca et al., in press].

Ritov and Baron [1989] have extended this demonstration in a study of decisions about hypothetical vaccination decisions. Subjects are reluctant to vaccinate a child when the vaccination itself can cause side effects as bad as the disease it prevents (even when these effects are much less likely). This effect is even greater when subjects are told of the existence of a 'risk group' for the side effects: If a child is in the risk group, the side effects are more likely, but if a child is not, the side effects will not occur, and a test for membership in the risk group is unavailable. This effect of ignorance is another kind of overgeneralization of a contingently relevant attribute. Ordinarily, it would be prudent to find out whether a child is in the risk group before acting, but in this case it is impossible, so knowledge of the existence of the risk group is irrelevant. (The overall probability is held constant, and the subject is told this.)

Sunk Cost and Endowment

In the sunk-cost effect [Arkes and Blumer, 1985; Thaler, 1980], subjects favor spending more resources on a project when they have already 'sunk' a lot of resources into it, even when they are told that such future expenditures can be more usefully deployed elsewhere. This effect, too, can be seen as an overgeneralization of the use of contingently relevant information. Specifically, the sunk-cost effect overgeneralizes a rule against waste. If your original decision were to put resources into a task that would not be completed, you would be foolish because you could use the resources better elsewhere. But when you have already sunk the resources, you cannot retrieve them to use elsewhere, and the rule against waste no longer serves its purpose. The irrelevant factor is loss compared to initial investment.

In addition, the sunk-cost heuristic attends to past expenditures. Ordinarily, past expenditures are an indicator of the wisdom of a decision. If I have put a lot of time and effort into a project, it is likely that I had good reason to do so. If I am unsure of whether to continue, past decisions are a good guide [Baron, 1988a, ch., 21]. But when the wisdom of continuing can be accurately assessed now, without relying on my past decisions, I ought to ignore the past. Such is the case in the laboratory studies of the sunk-cost effect [Arkes and Blumer, 1985]. Again, subjects overgeneralize a heuristic, possibly because they do not know its purpose and the arguments relating it to its purpose (particularly the fact that past decisions are generally well made).

Related phenomena are the endowment effect, in which subjects require more money to give up something than they are willing to pay for it [Knetsch and Sinden, 1984; Knetsch et al., 1988], and the status quo effect, in which subjects prefer the option they have (e.g., a retirement plan) to one they do not have, even though they regard the latter as superior when they have neither [Samuelson and Zeckhauser, 1988]. These effects could result from the same kind of overgeneralization that produces the sunk cost effect. When one has something, it is usually the result of having made a good decision. Or, in general, actions tend to make things worse rather than better, so we should 'leave well enough alone'. In the cases examined, however, these rationales do not apply because the future consequences of both options are equally well known.

Biases in Compensation

Another type of bias concerns the provision of compensation for misfortune. Compensation has several functions: It transfers money to those who need it most; it reduces envy by the unfortunate of the fortunate; it provides incentive to people to avoid hurting others or themselves; it provides retribution; and, finally, the knowledge that compensation is available reduces fear of uncompensated misfortune. The equalizing, fear-reducing, and envy-reducing functions apply regardless of whether the misfortune is caused by nature or by another person. The incentive and retribution functions apply only when the misfortune is caused by a person who can be made to suffer (e.g., by paying the compensation) as a result of causing the misfortune. Yet people judge that more compensation should be provided when harm is caused by people than when it is caused by nature, even when the incentive and retribution functions are removed [Ritov et al., 1989]. The removal of these functions was brought about by telling subjects that the victims never knew the cause of their accident, that the perpetrators never knew the effect of their carelessness on the victim (so that even the possibilities of reducing the victim's anger or making perpetrators feel guilty was held constant), that the provision of compensation was secret (so that no precedents were set), and that the compensation was provided from the estate of an eccentric multimillionaire, the sole purpose of which was to provide compensation (so that there was no question about the indirect responsibility of the donor for controlling the behavior of others).

This result appears to be a simple overgeneralization of a contingently relevant feature. Ordinarily, the compensation that is paid is correlated with the punishment that the perpetrator of the harm must suffer. In our examples, however, we have made the punishment of the perpetrator independent of the amount of compensation, so that punishment is no longer a relevant factor.

A second bias in compensation, perhaps related to the one just described, concerns the expectations of victims. Ritov et al. [1989] varied simultaneously the cause of an accident (human or mechanical) and the extent to which the accident might be 'abnormal'. A train accident in which a person is injured is caused either by the train running into a fallen tree (abnormal) or by the train's abrupt stop to avoid hitting the tree (normal, since the train was supposed to stop). The stop (or failure to stop) is caused either by the success or failure of a mechanical device or by the engineer's decision to stop or not. Subjects awarded more compensation to the victim (who does not know the cause of his misfortune) when the train failed to stop – the abnormal event – regardless of whether the failure was due to the machine or the engineer. This pattern of results concerning abnormal events seems to involve the overgeneralization of contingently relevant factors, since none of the factors is relevant in the cases we give. Specifically, when compensation provides an incentive to take precautions, this function is not served when precautions have been taken (when the train stopped). This is irrelevant here, because no incentive is provided. (The compensation was secret, etc.)

Belief in Moral Conventions as a Bias

Cultures teach morality in part by teaching rules such as the Ten Commandments. Most of these rules serve good purposes. The commandment against stealing prevents unexpected harm and supports the institution of property. The rule about honoring one's parents supports the institution of the family. In many cases, though, cultural rules could be changed without loss. Rules against calling teachers by their first names, for example, have been dropped in some schools without apparent ill effects. In the past, changes in rules have led to apparent improvements, such as in rules about slavery and about the rights of women.

We can think of 'breaking a cultural rule' then, as a contingently relevant factor in the judgment of immorality. The fact that a cultural rule is broken is a sign that an act is likely to lead to harm or weaken an important institution. But when we know the expected consequences of an act, we can judge for ourselves, putting aside the rule. Past generations made this sort of judgment about slavery and the subjugation of women. Some rules are more fundamental. We cannot think of how to establish a society without trying to enforce them. For example, the rule against hurting others solely for the purpose of one's own enrichment seems to be one we would always want to maintain. These sorts of moral rules serve as the justification for the kinds of conventions that can be justified in a particular society.

Turiel [1983] and his collaborators [Nucci, 1985] found that most children and adults in the USA and several other countries make a distinction between moral rules and conventional rules. They asked children whether it would be okay to call one's teacher by her first name if everyone thought it was okay, or to bow instead of shaking hands, or whether it would be okay for a bully to push another kid off the top of a slide if everyone thought it was okay. Even most second graders (age 7) said it would be okay to change the conventions but not the moral rules: It would still be wrong to push someone off of a slide, even if everyone thought it was not wrong.

Many children, however, fail to distinguish morality and convention. They think that it would be wrong to call a teacher by her first name, for a boy to come to class wearing a dress, or for children to take off their clothes at school if the weather got too hot, regardless of whether everyone thought it was wrong or not. Shweder et al. [1988] found such responses among adults and children in a Hindu village in India, and Jon Haidt [personal communication] has found that underprivileged children living in South America and the USA tend to make this sort of response most of the time, even for rules studied by Turiel. Haidt has also found that these children cannot explain why it would be wrong to change the conventions in terms of more fundamental moral principles. It seems that they would blindly follow the rule even if the conditions that make it applicable (its cultural context) were removed. They therefore overgeneralize the rule in the same way that many other rules are overgeneralized.

The Development of Biases

We might expect that children will at first learn rules relatively blindly and only later come to understand them. If this is so, biases should decrease with age or experience. Few studies have examined changes in biases as a result of experience. Some studies have found that biases that involve the misweighing of factors relative to one another are reduced with feedback [e.g., Camerer, 1987], but feedback is not our primary concern here. In many judgment situations – for example, those involving judgments of morality or long-term prudence – little or no feedback is available. Kuhn et al. [1988] have found that certain biases in hypothesis testing are reduced with experience, but we know little about the mechanism underlying these effects. Possibly what experience provides is the opportunity for thinking – for asking oneself about the purposes of a rule that one is following (search for goals), consideration of alternative possible rules, or search for evidence about whether a rule in fact serves its intended purposes.

Teubal et al. [1989] examined change in certain biases with age. We found very few age changes in recognition of the precedent-setting effects of decisions, the sunk-cost effect, the omission bias, or the use of probability as a guide to decisions (e.g., about wearing seatbelts). We did find differences between two groups of subjects, a group of mostly-Black inner-city children and adolescents attending a summer sports camp and a group of mostly-White gifted children attending a summer program for the gifted. Members of the sports group were more inclined to exhibit the sunk-cost effect and to ignore precedent setting, but they were less inclined to exhibit the omission bias. Although some biases can be affected by a general tendency to engage in actively open-minded thinking, it cannot account for the different patterns of results for the two groups. Specific cultural teaching undoubtedly plays some role. In our case, we speculated that the more religious upbringing of the sports group members had sensitized them to the moral issues in our omission-commission stories.

Biases can be reduced by specific types of education. Nisbett et al. [1987] examined the effects of various kinds of university instruction on statistical, logical, and methodological reasoning. Nisbett et al. found that logical reasoning improved as a result of two years of graduate school in law, medicine, or psychology. The largest improvement in statistical and methodological reasoning occurred among psychology students, probably because training in such things as the use of control groups is an important part of graduate work in psychology. Methodological reasoning also improved with medical training, which places some emphasis on the conduct and interpretation of medical research, but there was essentially no improvement from training in either law or chemistry.

These studies indicate that appropriate education in which certain methods of reasoning are explicitly emphasized can have general effects on the tendency to use these methods in everyday problems unrelated to the areas in which the methods were taught. They also suggest that some of these effects can be specific to particular reasoning methods. In particular, legal training affected logical but not statistical reasoning. What is not clear from these studies, however, is whether their results are applicable to the kinds of biases that have been discussed here and whether some of the observed improvement (particularly in psychology) might be attributable to increases in actively open-minded thinking.

Conclusion

These findings point to the importance of education in the reduction of biases. Biases do not seem to go away by themselves. If experience affords the opportunity to think about the rules we follow, then normal development does not provide much of the relevant experience. Without some sort of systematic cultural influences to the contrary, children may not show much spontaneous development of understanding of rules of judgment and decision-making of the sort that have been discussed here. In the course of history, of course, at least some people reflect on the reasons for things and attain certain insights. But for many of the rules we follow in daily life, it seems unlikely that each individual spontaneously discovers the insights achieved by great thinkers of the past. Adults must make an effort to pass on these insights to the young.

Education need not occur only in schools. Parents, as well as teachers, can discuss judgment rules with children. In doing this, they teach not only the purposes of specific rules but also the expectation that rules have purposes. Such an expectation leads both to an effort to understand and therefore respect the rules that we ask children to learn and to a healthy rebelliousness against rules that have no purpose.

Acknowledgements

I thank Jonathan Haidt for instruction about Turiel, and the National Science Foundation and National Institute of Mental Health for support of some of the research described here.

References

Arkes, H.R., & Blumer, C. (1985). The psychology of sunk cost. *Organizational Behavior and Human Decision Processes, 35,* 124–140.
Arkes, H.R., & Hammond, K.R. (1986). *Judgment and decision making: An interdisciplinary reader.* Cambridge: Cambridge University Press.
Baron, J. (1985). *Rationality and intelligence.* New York: Cambridge University Press.
Baron, J. (1986). Tradeoffs among reasons for action. *Journal for the Theory of Social Behavior, 16,* 173–195.
Baron, J. (1988a). *Thinking and deciding.* New York: Cambridge University Press.
Baron, J. (1988b). Utility, exchange, and commensurability. *Journal of Thought, 23,* 111–131.
Baron, J. (1989). Actively open-minded thinking versus myside bias: Causes and effect. Proceedings of the Fourth International Conference on Thinking, San Juan, 1989.
Baron, J. (in press). Beliefs about thinking. In J.F. Voss, D.N. Perkins, & J.W. Segal (Eds.), *Informal reasoning and education.* Hillsdale NJ: Erlbaum.
Baron, J. (in preparation). *Optimal goal achievement for self and others.*
Baron, J., & Hershey, J.C. (1988). Outcome bias in decision evaluation. *Journal of Personality and Social Psychology, 54,* 569–579.
Brehmer, B. (1980). In one word: Not from experience. *Acta Psychologica, 45,* 223–241.
Camerer, C. (1987). Do biases in probability judgment matter in markets? Experimental evidence. *American Economic Review, 77,* 981–997.
Christensen-Szalanski, J.J. (1978). Problem solving strategies: A selection mechanism, some implications and some data. *Organizational Behavior and Human Performance, 22,* 307–323.
Dershowitz, A. (1988). *New York Times,* May 29, sec. 4, p. 18.
Duncker, K. (1945). On problem solving. *Psychological Monographs, 58,* (Whole No. 270).
Frisch, D., & Baron, J. (1988). Ambiguity and rationality. *Journal of Behavioral Decision Making, 1,* 149–157.
Hare, R.M. (1981). *Moral thinking: Its levels, method and point.* Oxford: Oxford University Press.

Hoch, S.J. (1985). Counterfactual reasoning and accuracy in predicting personal events. *Journal of Experimental Psychology: Learning, Memory, and Cognition, 11*, 719–731.

Kahneman, D., Slovic, P., & Tversky, A. (Eds.) (1982). *Judgment under uncertainty: Heuristics and biases.* New York: Cambridge University Press.

Kahneman, D., & Tversky, A. (1984). Choices, values, and frames. *American Psychologist, 39*, 341–350.

Katona, G. (1940). *Organizing and memorizing: Studies in the psychology of learning and teaching.* New York: Columbia University Press.

Knetsch, J.L., & Sinden, J.A. (1984). Willingness to pay and compensation: Experimental evidence of an unexpected disparity in measures of value. *Quarterly Journal of Economics, 99*, 508–522.

Knetsch, J.L., Thaler, R.H., & Kahneman, D. (1988). *Experimental tests of the endowment effect and the Coase theorem.* Unpublished manuscript, Simon Fraser University.

Koriat, A., Lichtenstein, S., & Fischhoff, B. (1980). Reasons for confidence. *Journal of Experimental Psychology: Human Learning and Memory, 6*, 107–118.

Kuhn, D. (forthcoming). *The skills of argument.*

Kuhn, D., Amsel, E., & O'Loughlin, M. (1988). *The development of scientific thinking skills.* Orlando FL: Acadamic Press.

Larrick, R.P., Morgan J.N., & Nisbett, R.E. (1989). *Who uses the normative rules of choice?* Unpublished manuscript, University of Michigan.

Nickerson, R.S. (1989). On improving thinking through instruction. *Review of Research in Education, 15*, 3–57.

Nisbett, R.E., Fong, G.T., Lehman, D.R., & Cheng, P.W. (1987). Teaching reasoning. *Science, 238*, 625–631.

Nucci, L.P. (1985). Children's conceptions of morality, societal convention, and religious prescription. In C.G. Harding (Ed.), *Moral dilemmas: Philosophical and psychological issues in the development of moral reasoning* (pp. 137–174). Chicago: Precedent.

Paul, R.W. (1984). Critical thinking: Fundamental for education for a free society. *Educational Leadership, 42*, 4–14.

Payne, J.W., Bettman, J.R., & Johnson, E.J. (1988). Adaptive strategy selection in decision making. *Journal of Experimental Psychology: Learning, Memory and Cognition, 14*, 534–552.

Perkins, D.N. (1985). Postprimary education has little impact on informal reasoning. *Journal of Educational Psychology, 77*, 562–571.

Perkins, D.N. (1986). *Knowledge as design: Critical and creative thinking for teachers and learners.* Hillsdale NJ: Erlbaum.

Perkins, D.N. (in press). Reasoning as it is and could be: An empirical perspective. In D. Topping, D. Crowell, & V. Kobayashi (Eds.), *Thinking: The third international conference.* Hillsdale NJ: Erlbaum.

Perkins, D.N., Bushey, B., & Faraday, M. (1986). *Learning to reason.* Unpublished manuscript, Harvard University.

Ritov, I., Hodes, J., & Baron, J. (1989). *Biases in decisions about compensation for misfortune.* Unpublished manuscript, University of Pennsylvania.

Ritov, I., & Baron, J. (1989). *Reluctance to vaccinate: Commission bias and ambiguity.* Unpublished manuscript, University of Pennsylvania.

Samuelson, W., & Zeckhauser, R. (1988). Status quo bias in decision making. *Journal of Risk and Uncertainty, 1,* 7–59.

Schoenfeld, A.H. (1985). *Mathematical problem solving.* New York: Academic Press.

Shweder, R.A., Mahapatra, M., & Miller, J.G. (1988). Culture and moral development. In J. Kagan (Ed.), *The emergence of moral concepts in young children* (pp. 1–83). Chicago: University of Chicago Press.

Spranca, M., Minsk, E., & Baron, J. (in press). Omission and commission in judgment and choice. *Journal of Experimental Social Psychology.*

Teubal, E., Spranca, M., & Baron, J. (1989). *Decision-making biases in children and adolescents: Exploratory studies.* Unpublished manuscript, University of Pennsylvania.

Thaler, R. (1985). Mental accounting and consumer choice. *Marketing Science, 4,* 199–214.

Turiel, E. (1983). *The development of social knowledge: Morality and convention.* New York: Cambridge University Press.

Wertheimer, M. (1959). *Productive thinking* (rev. ed.). New York: Harper & Row. (Original work published 1945.)

Kuhn D (ed): Developmental Perspectives on Teaching and Learning Thinking Skills.
Contrib Hum Dev. Basel, Karger, 1990, vol 21, pp 48–62

A Skill Approach to the Development of Reflective Thinking

Karen Strohm Kitchener, Kurt W. Fischer

Educators at all levels have claimed that one of the central aims of education is the development of judgment, reflective thinking, and similar higher-order thought processes [Kitchener, 1983]. Because of the importance of these skills, many institutions of higher education have established courses designed to teach them, usually under the rubric of critical thinking [McMillen, 1986]. Although educators frequently give lip service to the breadth of skills involved in critical thinking, most often the skills are defined and taught narrowly – as logical reasoning, following the principles of deductive logic [Brabeck, 1983]. In addition, most educators and researchers have taken a traditional learning theory approach, portraying the acquisition of these skills as occurring via a gradual accumulation of learned behavior or rules [Glaser, 1941; Kitchener, 1983; Klahr and Wallace, 1976]. Development has been described primarily in environmental terms involving conditioning or other learning mechanisms.

We take issue with both of these assumptions. First, we argue that logic is insufficient to characterize higher-order reasoning about all problems. Instead, assumptions about knowledge play a crucial role, particularly in ill-structured problem solving. A useful way of analyzing these assumptions is through the reflective judgment model, which describes the development of knowledge assumptions [Kitchener, 1986; Kitchener and King, 1981]. Second, we suggest that an interactional approach is required to understand the development of thinking skills. Development can be adequately understood only through analysis of how the person and the environment collaborate in development [Fischer and Bullock, in press]. Learning approaches focusing primarily on environmental influences neglect the developing person.

To cast the development of critical thinking in an interactive or collaborational framework, we describe a model of the development of reflective judgment based on skill theory [Fischer, 1980]. This model leads to a conception of development that characterizes both the levels of development of a person's thinking and the range of variations in levels that each person normally shows. This developmental analysis of reflective judgment has important implications for education in critical or higher-order thinking.

The Nature of Higher-Order Reasoning Skills

It has been difficult to define higher-order reasoning or critical thinking [Skinner, 1976], but there appears to be some consensus about the class of skills involved. An analysis we have found especially useful is Dewey's [1933]. Central to his concept of reflective thinking, which he also called problem solving, critical thinking, and reflective judgment, is the understanding that such thinking is needed in truly problematic situations, ones in which there is real uncertainty. In fact, work on critical thinking has been hampered by a failure to acknowledge the importance of situations of real uncertainty.

Problems vary in the degree to which they can be solved with certainty [Kitchener, 1983]. 'Well-structured' problems can be defined with a high degree of completeness and solved with a high degree of certainty [Churchman, 1971; Wood, 1983]. The parameters of the problem are specified or knowable. Single correct answers exist that can be verified by others such as experts or by the appropriate use of an algorithm, formula, or other effective procedure. Problems of deductive logic fall into this category.

Other problems, called 'ill-structured' or 'wicked-decision' problems [Churchman, 1971], cannot be described with a high degree of completeness nor solved with certainty. Real-life problems, such as what to do about overpopulation or how to predict the likelihood of the greenhouse effect, have unknown or unknowable parameters. Solutions must be constructed using evidence, expert opinion, reason, and argument, but no effective procedure is available that can guarantee a correct solution. In other words, logic alone is insufficient to generate and construct solutions.

Kitchener and King [1981; 1990] have argued that the ability to construct reasonable solutions for ill-structured problems is dependent upon developmental changes in epistemological assumptions. They point out

Table 1. Relation between skill levels and reflective judgment stages

Reflective judgment stage: Nature of knowledge, justification	Type of behavior	Skill level
Stage 1 What a person believes to be true is true. No justification is necessary.	Knowing is limited to concrete instances, such as A; e.g., I know there is cereal in the box.	Level Rp 1 Single representation: concrete instance of knowing. [A]
Stage 2 A person can know with certainty either directly or via an authority.	Right answers about A (A_R) are contrasted with wrong answers about A (A_W).	Level Rp 2 Representational mapping, which coordinates concrete representations with each other. [$A_R - A_W$]
Justification is via an authority.	Right answers about A are justified by Authority X's answer to A (A_X).	[$A_R - A_X$]
Stage 3 In some areas knowledge is temporarily uncertain: Justification is based on what feels right at the moment.	In areas that are temporarily uncertain, Authorities V and W, who both know about C, endorse different conclusions S and T ($C_{S,V}$ and $C_{T,W}$).	Level Rp 3 Representational system, in which several aspects of two concrete representations are coordinated. [$C_{S,V} \longleftrightarrow C_{T,W}$]
In other areas, authorities truly know, and knowledge is certain.	In areas known for sure, Authority X knows the right answer about A ($A_{R,X}$), and Authority Y knows the right answer about B ($B_{R,Y}$).	[$A_{R,X} \longleftrightarrow B_{R,Y}$]

Stage		Level
Stage 4 Knowledge is generally uncertain because of situational variables. What we know and how we justify beliefs is idiosyncratic.	Abstract conception that any item of knowledge, K, is uncertain. What we can know about A and B varies in different authorities X and Y as a function of situations P and Q of the authorities.	**Level Rp 4 – A 1** System of representational systems, which is the same as a single abstraction. $$\begin{bmatrix} A_{P,X} \leftrightarrow A_{Q,Y} \\ \updownarrow \\ B_{P,X} \leftrightarrow B_{Q,Y} \end{bmatrix} = [K]$$
Stage 5 Knowledge is contextual: People know via individual conceptual filters. Justification is context-specific.	Each (uncertain) item of knowledge, K, can be justified by a particular argument, J, in a context F.	**Level A 2**[a] Abstract mapping, which coordinates abstractions with each other. $[K_F — J_F]$
Stage 6 Knowledge is constructed by comparing evidence and opinion on different sides of an issue or across contexts. Justification involves explaining such comparisons.	Each item of knowledge can be justified by evidence from several contexts or sides of an issue, F and G.	**Level A 3** Abstract system, in which several aspects of two abstractions are coordinated. $[K_{F,G} \leftrightarrow J_{F,G}]$
Stage 7 Knowledge is an outcome of an inquiry process that is generalizable across issues. Justification is probabilistic, involving the use of evidence and argument to present the most complete or compelling understanding of an issue.	General principle that knowing is the outcome of the process of justifying and defending beliefs: Comparisons of justifications, J and N, for differing arguments, K and M, across several contexts, F and G or H and I, lead to a conclusion about the argument that is most probably true.	**Level A 4** System of abstract systems, which is the same as a single principle. $$\begin{bmatrix} K_{F,G} \leftrightarrow J_{F,G} \\ \updownarrow \\ M_{H,I} \leftrightarrow N_{H,I} \end{bmatrix}$$

The skills specified for each stage are typical of that stage, but they are not exhaustive: There can be other skills with similar structures and different contents. In the skill formulas, italic capital letters designate representational sets, and large capital letters designate abstract sets. Multiple subscripts designate differentiated components of a set. Long straight lines and arrows designate a relation between sets or systems. Brackets designate a single skill.

[a] Representational structures continue at later levels of abstractions, but the formulas become too complex if all components are shown. To fill in the representational structures, simply replace each abstract set with a representational formula similar to that for Level Rp 4.

that certain assumptions are incompatible with ill-structured problem solving. For example, the belief that absolute knowledge can be attained presumes that problem solutions are certain and that the problem solver's task is to identify the correct one. It precludes the possibility that problem parameters are unknowable or that solutions must be practically constructed.

Unlike those who suggest that higher-order reasoning skills result only from the accumulation of learned skills, Kitchener and King have argued that the epistemic assumptions on which ill-structured problem solving rests develop through seven stages or levels. These levels are qualitatively different forms of justification, each of which characterizes a distinct approach to the development and defense of beliefs about ill-structured problems. In other words, the nature of the judgment process, what is admitted as evidence, and how evidence is synthesized into a viewpoint is qualitatively different at each stage.

In early stages individuals hold concrete concepts of knowing (table 1, left-hand column). They believe that real problems that presume uncertainty do not exist, and so they have little need for justification beyond reference to authorities. In the middle stages, people begin to understand that uncertainty is a fundamental aspect of knowing, but they are unable to move beyond their own idiosyncratic views in the justification of beliefs. In the later stages, people acknowledge the uncertainty of knowing, but they also argue that knowledge is an outcome of an inquiry process based on probabilistic justification. The form of reasoning in these later stages is similar to what Dewey characterized as reflective thinking and seems to us to describe an essential aspect of what educators often mean by critical thinking.

Research has supported the predictions of the model. The seven stages develop in the predicted sequence, according to both longitudinal and cross-sectional tests of sequentiality [Davison et al., 1980]. The reflective judgment scores of secondary and post-secondary students consistently increase with age and educational level [Kitchener and King, 1990]. Across studies, mean stage scores have ranged from 2.8 to 3.3 for high school students, 3.4 to 4.0 for undergraduate students, and 4.2 to 5.4 for graduate students. In the four longitudinal studies that have been completed to date, the age changes found were similar to the age differences identified in cross-sectional studies.

Although the reflective judgment model characterizes development in terms of seven stages, the data collected so far have shown gradual development, with no clear spurts or plateaus for stage acquisition, as some would predict [Fischer and Kenny, 1986]. The new skill model addresses this issue. Another issue that is addressed by the skill model is how environmental factors contribute to stage change. For example, several studies have shown that formal educational experience plays an important role in the development of reflective judgment, a role that goes beyond the effects of age by itself [Glatfelter, 1982; Lawson, 1980; Kitchener et al., 1989; Schmidt, 1985; Shoff, 1979; Strange and King, 1981]. Prior work has not addressed the specific processes underlying such effects but has been limited to a global Piagetian framework, which assumes interaction of person and environment without specifying much about the nature of the interaction. The one thing that has been specified is the hypothesis that the promotion of reflective judgment requires an environment that emphasizes what one can know, how one can know, and the need for judgment even in light of uncertainty [Kitchener et al., 1989]. With its focus on both person and environment, the skill model shifts the emphasis to how a person's stage varies as a function of environmental factors. Previous work used global stage descriptions to characterize a person's thinking, but the new approach focuses on the normal range of variation for an individual.

Key Ideas in Skill Theory

Skill theory is designed to provide a fuller picture of development by considering the collaboration of the developing person and the environment in which a behavior occurs [Fischer, 1980]. It assumes that developmental level cannot be accurately measured or understood without taking into consideration characteristics of both the person and the environment, including the immediate context of a behavior. With its focus on variation in level, it also explains how developmental patterns change with assessment condition. For example, behavior both develops in a stage-like way and also demonstrates slow, continuous change, depending on the condition. In the same way, the level of behavior can be both consistent and variable across contexts.

According to skill theory, there are two types of processes that produce development [Fischer and Pipp, 1984]. The process of optimal level explains the major cognitive changes that people show over a long period of time. The process of skill acquisition describes how people learn specific skills both between and within levels.

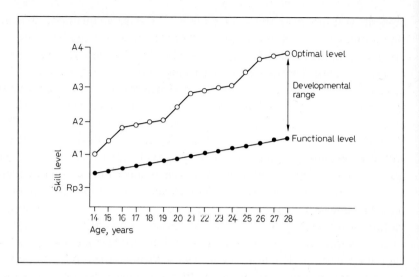

Fig. 1. Idealized growth curves for developmental range in adolescence and early adulthood.

Optimal level is defined as the upper limit of the person's general information processing capacity, i.e., the most complex type of skill that the person can control. While individual performance may vary widely across contexts, it does not exceed an optimal level of complexity. As optimal level increases with age, the change is not linear but stage-like – spurts alternating with plateaus in growth as illustrated by the upper line in figure 1.

Each period of spurts marks the emergence of a new developmental level characterized by a qualitatively different skill structure. A person's best performance in a familiar domain improves sharply when a new level is emerging. For the age period shown in figure 1, the spurt in optimal performance is followed by a period of several years during which optimal performance increases slowly, in a growth plateau. These plateaus do not indicate developmental stasis but instead mark a time of extension and elaboration of skills. It is only optimal performance that shows such limited growth.

Seven optimal skill levels are hypothesized to emerge between 2 and 30 years of age [Fischer and Farrar, 1987]. According to the skill model, these seven levels relate directly to the seven stages of reflective judgment. Each reflective judgment stage can be accomplished for the first time at the skill level shown in table 1. (We will not discuss the six additional levels that according to skill theory emerge in the first two years.) During the years of childhood, the skills that emerge involve concrete representations of people, objects, or events. With the emergence of each new level, children are able to construct more complex relations between concrete representations. At these skill levels, which are hypothesized to constitute the first three stages of reflective judgement, the representations of knowledge are concrete. At the first representational level, individuals can work only with single concrete representations about what they know. At the second level, they can relate two concrete representations to each other, such as what two authorities know. The third level allows for understanding more complex relations between different authorities and the domains they know.

By the fourth level, representations are related in complex combinations that produce a new kind of thinking, single abstractions, which forms the first of four abstract levels. In a single abstraction about knowledge, a person coordinates concrete knowledge about how different people draw different conclusions, based on their own circumstances or 'biases'. From this coordination emerges the abstraction that knowledge is uncertain. As with representations, single abstractions are then related to each other to form the fifth level; here an abstract justification can be related to an item of knowledge in an abstract mapping. At the sixth level, individuals can form abstract systems, in which several sides or contexts for justification of a knowledge item are coordinated. Finally, at the seventh level, individuals develop systems of abstract systems, in which two or more abstract systems are related to form a principle. With respect to reflective judgment, one principle is that knowledge is the outcome of a general inquiry process that can produce compelling, highly probable conclusions.

Although optimal level specifies the upper limit in the complexity of skill that an individual can control, actual functioning at the upper limit requires that performance be induced and supported by the environment. Practice, task difficulty, and procedure are all related to performance. Thus, only under optimal environmental conditions – when individuals have had an opportunity to master a skill and there is contextual support for high-level performance – are the spurts in performance that indicate the emergence of a new level uniformly evident. Under these conditions, people demonstrate stage-like development in a variety of domains.

Skill acquisition, the second type of process involved in skill theory, describes how a person learns or acquires individual skills. These processes determine how specific skills are constructed, including how the person moves from a particular skill in a given context to a more complex or general skill. These processes are defined by a set of transformation rules, which specify how particular skills are transformed to form new skills. The individual acquiring or generalizing a skill proceeds through a microdevelopmental sequence involving many small steps specified by the rules. The reflective judgment stages capture only large jumps between levels, not these smaller microdevelopmental steps.

Under ordinary circumstances, skill development proceeds slowly and somewhat haphazardly, showing the slow, gradual change illustrated by the lower line in figure 1. At any one time, life events may or may not place two skills in relation to each other in the person's experience. When the juxtaposition does occur, it leads the person to work out a coordination of the skills, transforming them into new ones. In addition, the environment does not often provide cues or support for high-level performance. As a result, people typically perform not at their optimal level, but at their lower, functional level. Improvement in functional level usually is slow and gradual, with performance remaining far below optimal level and varying widely across domains. However, performance improves dramatically as soon as contextual support is provided for optimal performance [Fischer and Bullock, in press].

Researchers have found repeatedly that individual performance varies under different testing conditions and in diverse domains [Biggs and Collis, 1982; Fischer, 1980; Flavell, 1982]. The difference between optimal and functional level is responsible for much of this variation. For a given person in a given content domain this difference is called the developmental range, as shown in figure 1. The concept of developmental range leads beyond standard characterizations of the individuals' thinking in terms of a point on a developmental scale. In assessments and interventions, researchers and teachers need to assume that individuals can operate within a range of stages or levels, depending centrally on the amount of contextual support provided for high-level performance.

Functional and Optimal Levels of Reflective Judgment

Reflective judgment has been measured by the Reflective Judgment Interview (RJI), in which people are asked to form a judgment about an ill-structured problem that is described from at least two opposing viewpoints, such as whether chemical additives to food are helpful or dangerous. They then are asked to explain their rationale for that judgment. The skill model predicts that development as assessed by the RJI will appear slow and gradual, as it has in previous research. The RJI assesses functional level because it does not provide optimal contextual support for performance. Also, it tests people in domains with which they may be only generally familiar. In this way, it is similar to many other developmental measures such as Loevinger's [1976] sentence completion test, Kohlberg's moral judgment interview [Colby and Kohlberg, 1987], and Damon and Hart's [1988] self interview.

Fischer has suggested two procedures that facilitate the study of how person and environment interact to produce developmental level [Fischer and Kenny, 1986]. First, an independent assessment for each step in the developmental sequence provides a powerful measure of the sequence and allows for more precision in testing hypotheses. Second, the research design should vary both person characteristics, such as age and gender, and environmental conditions. In recent research, a new instrument, the Prototypic Reflective Judgment Interview (PRJ), was devised to meet both of these criteria and thereby evaluate both optimal and functional levels in reflective judgment. This instrument was inspired in part by early work by Rest [1973] on moral judgment.

In the PRJ, people are given two of the ill-structured problems used in the RJI (on chemical additives and building of the pyramids). Contextual support is provided by presentation of a prototypic answer for each stage for each problem [Kitchener et al., 1989]. The prototypic answers are based on real responses of people to these problems on the RJI. For each stage of each problem, the participant is asked to read one of the statements. The interviewer then poses a series of questions that direct attention to key aspects of the statement. Finally, participants are asked to explain the meaning of the statement in their own words. Explanations are scored 'hit' if the participant gives a consistent, accurate summary of the prototypic statement, and 'miss' if not. The same procedure is repeated for each of the prototypic statements for reflective judgment stages 2 to 7 for both problems.

Participants in a recent study of the PRJ were 104 students between 14 and 28 years of age, half male and half female. They were tested individually in two sessions two weeks apart. During each session, the students first responded to the RJI, as a measure of functional level, and then to the PRJ, a high-support measure designed to move performance toward optimal level. After the first session, participants were also given two good examples of reflective judgment reasoning, one at the highest stage 'hit' during the first session, as well as one at the next highest stage. These examples did not make direct reference to the issues of chemical additives or pyramids. Thus, during the second session participants were tested after some practice and instruction, and once again the PRJ provided high contextual support. The PRJ at the second session therefore provided the best estimate of optimal level.

Although the results are too numerous to be reported in detail, three general findings are important for the present discussion: (1) As predicted, nearly all students performed better in the high-support conditions than in the low-support ones. While scores on the spontaneous measure (RJI) replicated results of previous studies for each age level, scores on the high-support measure (PRJ) were significantly higher. The difference in performance as a function of the two testing conditions remained similar at the second session, after students had the opportunity for practice. While the scores on both measures increased modestly, the gap remained. (2) An age-related ceiling was evident in the high-support condition (PRJ) even after practice, as predicted by the optimal-level hypothesis. For example, students younger than 19 did not effectively explain Stage 6 statements, but many students 20 years of age and older did explain them well. (3) In the high-support condition there was evidence of an age-related developmental spurt with each stage. For example, for Stage 6, no students were able to pass the tasks at age 18 and earlier, but 50% or more passed them at age 20 and beyond.

The results of this study suggest that students typically operate at one developmental level when they act spontaneously (without contextual support) and at a higher developmental level when they experience contextual support and practice. In other words, reflective judgment performance can best be characterized by a developmental range. Furthermore, the results indicate that optimal development in reflective judgment can be characterized by a spurt followed by a plateau in performance for each reflective judgment stage. Earlier skill-theory research has shown similar developmental patterns with arithmetic as well as other tasks [Fischer and Lamborn, 1989].

These results capture an important part of the naturally occurring variation in reflective thinking, but it is important to recognize that there is additional variation as well. The nature of the ill-defined problem and the person's background can affect stage score. For example, Kitchener et al. [1989] report that in response to four standard RJI problems, students' modal score was consistent on three of the four problems while on the fourth it was discrepant by one or more stages.

Educational Implications of the Skill Approach

As noted at the outset, educators at all levels have identified 'critical thinking' as a major goal of education. Often critical thinking involves making and defending complex judgments about ill-structured problems. According to the reflective judgment model, the ability to make such judgments depends on the emergence of the epistemic assumptions that characterize Stages 6 and 7. Data from the study we just described suggest that even with contextual support, practice, and instruction, students under the ages of 19 or 20 cannot consistently understand such concepts well enough to explain them in their own words. Of course, it is probable that more practice and support would have led to further advance, but we predict that the primary result would be that more students would perform at the highest stage their age mates already show rather than moving beyond to later stages. For example, 16 year olds would become more skilled at making Stage 5 arguments, but they would still struggle with Stage 6 and 7 arguments.

According to skill theory, skills are hard to learn and sustain, with the result that in most domains, performance often occurs below optimal level even when assessed under high-support conditions and with the opportunity for practice [Fischer and Bullock, in press]. Movement to optimal level requires sustained work at mastering and internalizing the skills. Educational systems, which tend to emphasize solving of well-structured problems, seldom provide high levels of instruction or contextual support for the upper levels of reflective judgment. Consequently, the person seldom experiences the pairing of inconsistent lower-level reflective judgment skills; in other words, people are not confronted with the contradictions. It is when this pairing occurs that the person has an opportunity to work out new higher-level coordinations. For example, when contradictions regarding ill-structured problems co-occur in an essay, instructors can highlight the discrepancy. When teachers focus instead on well-structured problems, students are not given the opportunity to carry out the hard work that is necessary to understand the bases of knowledge about ill-structured problems. The result is slow movement toward higher stages.

Without major changes in classroom emphasis from well-structured problems to ill-structured ones, as well as direct emphasis on the nature of the knowing process itself, it is unlikely that even college freshmen, much less high school or elementary school students, will be able to use or understand critical thinking as a process of inquiry applied to solving ill-structured problems. If such a change in emphasis did occur, students could build much more sophisticated reflective thinking skills than are currently typical. They probably would not be able to reach the highest stages of reflective judgment until their 20s, but they could develop deep understandings at the lower and middle stages. Reasoning about argument and justification are complex and interesting at these earlier stages too, and these skills lay the foundations for rapid development of reflective thinking at the later stages.

In applying the skill approach to education, it is crucial to remember that most classroom behavior – and most behavior in everyday life – involves performance at functional levels far below optimal level. Educators need to target not only optimal performance, but ordinary performance. If the goal is to produce sophisticated reflective thinking, students can learn to function near their optimum in some domains. For those skills, students' functional level will nearly equal their optimum. It is probably not possible – nor even desirable – for people to function at their optimum level in everything they do. But in areas that are worthy of a major educational effort, such as reflective thinking, it should be possible to have the two developmental lines in figure 1 nearly converge.

It is ordinary, functional performance that is most likely to affect students' daily lives in the real world outside the classroom. Talented teachers can undoubtedly produce high-support conditions in the classroom to promote optimal performance, and that is a good start. But they then need to go beyond those optimal conditions to help students produce the same sophisticated arguments on their own, without the support. A major goal of future research on reflective thinking should be to uncover methods of promoting students' functional levels of reflective judgment.

Acknowledgements

Preparation of this article was supported by grants from the Spencer Foundation and Harvard University. We would like to thank Cindy Lynch for her contributions to the arguments presented here.

References

Biggs, J., & Collis, K. (1982). *Evaluating the quality of learning: The SOLO taxonomy (structure of the observed learning outcome).* New York: Academic Press.

Brabeck, M. (1983). Critical thinking skills and reflective judgment development: Redefining the aims of higher education. *Journal of Applied Developmental Psychology, 4,* 23–34.

Churchman, C.W. (1971). *The design of inquiring systems: Basic concepts of systems and organizations.* New York: Basic Books.

Colby, A., & Kohlberg, L. (1987). *The measurement of moral judgment* (2 vols.). New York: Cambridge University Press.

Damon, W., & Hart, D. (1988). *Self-understanding in childhood and adolescence.* New York: Cambridge University Press.

Davison, M.L., King, P.M., Kitchener, K.S., & Parker, C.A. (1980). The stage sequence concept in cognitive social development. *Developmental Psychology, 16,* 121–131.

Dewey, J. (1933). *How we think.* New York: D.C. Heath.

Fischer, K.W. (1980). A theory of cognitive development: The control and construction of hierarchies of skills. *Psychological Review, 87,* 477–531.

Fischer, K.W., & Bullock, D. (in press). The failure of competence: How context contributes directly to skill. In R. Wozniak & K.W. Fischer (Eds.), *Specific environments: Thinking in contexts. Jean Piaget Society Series on Knowledge and Development.* Hillsdale NJ: Erlbaum.

Fischer, K.W., & Farrar, M.J. (1987). Generalizations about generalization: How a theory of skill development explains both generality and specificity. *International Journal of Psychology, 22,* 643–677.

Fischer K.W., & Kenny, S.L. (1986). The environmental conditions for discontinuities in the development of abstractions. In R. Mines & K. Kitchener (Eds.), *Adult cognitive development: Methods and models* (pp. 57–75). New York: Praeger.

Fischer, K.W., & Lamborn, S. (1989). Mechanisms of variation in developmental levels: Cognitive and emotional transitions during adolescence. In A. de Ribaupierre (Ed.), *Transition mechanisms in child development* (pp. 33–67). New York: Cambridge University Press.

Fischer, K.W., & Pipp, S.L. (1984). Processes of cognitive development: Optimal level and skill acquisition. In R.J. Sternberg (Ed.), *Mechanisms of cognitive development* (pp. 45–80). New York: Freeman.

Flavell, J. (1982). On cognitive development. *Child Development, 53,* 1–10.

Glaser, E.M. (1941). *An experiment in the development of critical thinking.* New York: Bureau of Publications, Teachers College, Columbia University.

Glatfelter, M. (1982). Identity development, intellectual development, and their relationship in reentry women students. (Doctoral dissertation, University of Minnesota). *Dissertation Abstracts International, 43.* 354A.

Kitchener, K.S. (1983). Cognition, metacognition, and epistemic cognition: A three-level model of cognitive processing. *Human Development, 4,* 222–232.

Kitchener, K.S. (1986). The reflective judgment model: Characteristics, evidence, and measurement: In R.A. Mines & K.S. Kitchener (Eds.), *Cognitive development in young adults.* New York: Praeger.

Kitchener, K.S., & King, P.M. (1981). Reflective judgment: Concepts of justification and their relationship to age and education. *Journal of Applied Developmental Psychology*, 2, 89–116.

Kitchener, K.S., & King, P.M. (1990). The reflective judgment model: Ten years of research. In M.L. Commons, C. Armon, L. Kohlberg, F.A. Richards, T.A. Grotzer, & J.D. Sinnott (Eds.), *Adult development 3: Models and methods in the study of adolescent and adult thought.* New York: Praeger.

Kitchener, K.S., King, P.M., Wood, P.K., & Davison, M.L. (1989). Sequentiality and consistency in the development of Reflective Judgment: A six year longitudinal study. *Journal of Applied Developmental Psychology, 10,* 73–95.

Kitchener, K.S., Lynch, C.L., & Fischer, K.W. (1989). A skill theory approach to the assessment of Reflective Judgment. Paper presented at the American Psychological Association annual meeting, New Orleans.

Klahr, D., & Wallace, J.G. (1976). *Cognitive development: An information-processing view.* Hillsdale NJ: Erlbaum.

Lamborn, S.D., & Fischer, K.W. (1988). Optimal and functional levels in cognitive development: The individual's developmental range. *Newsletter of the International Society for the Study of Behavioral Development,* No. 2 (Serial No. 14), 1–4.

Lawson, J.M. (1980). The relationship between graduate education and the development of reflective judgment: A function of age or educational experience. (Doctoral dissertation, University of Minnesota). *Dissertation Abstracts International, 41,* 4655A.

Loevinger, J. (1976). *Ego development: Concepts and theories.* San Francisco: Jossey-Bass.

McMillen, L. (March, 1986). Many professors now start at the beginning by teaching their students how to think. *The Chronical of Higher Education,* pp. 23 and 25.

Rest, J.R. (1973). The hierarchical nature of moral judgment: A study of patterns of comprehension. *Journal of Personality and Social Psychology, 41,* 86–109.

Schmidt, J.A. (1985). Older and wiser? A longitudinal study of the impact of college on intellectual development. *Journal of College Student Personnel, 26,* 388–394.

Shoff, S.P. (1979). The significance of age, sex, and type of education on the development of reasoning in adults. (Doctoral dissertation, University of Utah). *Dissertation Abstracts International, 40,* 3910A.

Skinner, S.B. (1976). Cognitive development: A prerequisite for critical thinking. *The Clearing House, 49,* 292–299.

Strange, C.C., & King, P.M. (1981). Intellectual development and its relationship to maturation during the college years. *Journal of Applied Developmental Psychology, 2,* 281–295.

Wood, P.K. (1983). Inquiring systems and problem structure: Implications for cognitive development. *Human Development, 26,* 249–265.

Kuhn D (ed): Developmental Perspectives on Teaching and Learning Thinking Skills.
Contrib Hum Dev. Basel, Karger, 1990, vol 21, pp 63–78

Teaching Thinking Skills:
We're Getting the Context Wrong

Lynn Okagaki, Robert J. Sternberg

To say that context affects cognition is to say nothing new. Many have
sounded the contextualist horn. Why, then, when we look at curriculum
designed to teach thinking skills – skills that obviously fall within the cognitive domain – do we find little, if any, consideration of contextual factors? In this chapter, we propose that context affects the development and
teaching of thinking skills in two distinct ways. First, it means that a child
does not come to the classroom as a 'tabula rasa'. Rather, environmental
factors outside the classroom will affect the development of thinking skills
and, therefore, will affect children's classroom performance. Second, it
means that thinking skills are learned in context, and the skills become
'contextualized'. That is, there are a variety of environmental elements
that become part of that skill use and make transfer of the skill to different
contexts difficult. When thinking skills are taught in school, the school
setting will have a contextualizing effect on the development of those
thinking skills. However, the school context may, in fact, be the wrong
context for developing widely applied thinking skills.

In this chapter we first define context and identify four types of effects
that context has on the development of thinking skills. Second, we propose
a model for considering the impact of one contextual influence – parental
beliefs – on the development of children's thinking. Third, we argue that
the contextualizing effect of school on the development of thinking skills
limits the applicability of these thinking skills. Finally, we propose ways to
make school a better context for the development of thinking skills.

Context Matters

This chapter is based on the premise that intellectual development is not solely a function of internal factors, but is also a function of one's context. Several psychologists have argued for the importance of context in cognition [Gelman, 1978; Goodnow, 1976; Luria, 1976; Neisser, 1976; Rogoff, 1982]. In this section, we define what we mean by 'context' and then briefly describe four effects that context has on the development of thinking skills. For comprehensive reviews of contextualist perspectives, see chapters by the Laboratory of Comparative Human Cognition [1982] and Rogoff [1982].

Defining Context

Broadly speaking, an individual's context consists of the 'structures and processes in both the immediate and more remote environment [that shape] the course of human development throughout the lifespan' [Bronfenbrenner, 1979, p. 11]. Accordingly, we are concerned with both the individual's physical environment (e.g., climate, physical structures, amount of space, types of objects and resources in the environment) and social environment (e.g., the roles, behaviors, and activities that occur in a particular setting). Specifically, we want to consider: (a) the immediate setting in which the individual is participating (e.g., the home, the school, a post office, or a playground), (b) the relation between the immediate setting and other settings in which the individual participates (e.g., the relation between the individual's home and school environments or home and work environments), and (c) the larger cultural context in which the individual lives [Bronfenbrenner, 1977, 1979]. Given this definition of context, how does context affect the development of thinking skills? What parameters are set when a thinking skill is learned in a particular context?

Contextual Effects

First, the immediate context provides specific objects upon which to act and defines the ways in which these objects are used. Reasoning with one set of objects is not necessarily the same as reasoning with a different set of objects. For example, in a study of rural, unschooled and schooled Indian children and American school children, Lantz [1979] found that a simple change from thinking about one set of objects (an array of colors) to thinking about a different set of objects (an array of grains and seeds) dramatically affected performance on a classification task. Similarly, the way an object is used in one setting can affect the way it is used in a different setting [Laboratory of Comparative Human Cognition, 1982].

A second way in which the immediate environment affects cognition is by giving supportive cues for practical problem solving. An example of the supportive effect of the physical environment is found in recent work by Scribner [1984, 1986] on practical or everyday problem solving. Her analyses of the on-the-job problem-solving strategies of dairy workers suggest that practical problem solving is dependent upon or supported by the environment. With the seeming strategy of finding the least-effort solution (mental or physical), workers automatically converted the multiplication required on a delivery ticket (e.g., '17 quarts skim milk @ 0.68 per quart') to a simpler problem (e.g., '1 case skim milk @ 10.88 plus 1 quart @ 0.68). The conversion is 'suggested' by the environment in which the worker is physically delivering one case (which consists of 16 quarts) plus one additional quart. Everyday problem solving is often serendipitous, and requires active involvement with one's context.

Third, when thinking skills are learned in particular contexts, expectations about appropriate behaviors, response choices, and social roles are also established, and these expectations can become part of the supporting context that the child sees as necessary for implementing that skill. When the behaviors and expectations in one setting do not sufficiently match those of another setting or context, then, although the skill may be present, the individual may be confused as to what is being required of him or her. In an ethnographic study of three communities in the Piedmont Carolinas, Heath [1983] described a community in which children are rarely asked to answer questions from adults. Children do not take the role of information-givers. Heath suggests that, as a result, these children are confused when they are constantly asked to respond to questions from adults in school – particularly when the adults already know the answers to the questions. The children may, in fact, know the answers to the questions, but the school context is not giving them the necessary cues to enable children to know that they are supposed to say what they know.

Finally, the cultural context in which thinking skills are learned sets the criteria for what is accepted as a 'good' answer or as 'good thinking'. For example, Cole et al. [1971] presented Kpelle farmers with a set of 20 items, five each from four categories – food, clothing, tools, and cooking utensils. The subjects were asked to sort the objects into groups of objects that go together. Instead of putting objects into the four taxonomic categories, the Kpelle subjects, for example, put the potato with the pot. After all, one needs the pot to cook the potato. Subjects indicated that a wise man would put things together in this manner. Finally, when the experimenters asked how a fool would do the task, they got the answer they originally expected. Obviously, the Kpelle did have the ability to do the taxonomic classification, but a taxonomic classification was not a sensible response, according to Kpelle standards.

In sum, the context in which thinking skills develop: (a) dictates what objects and ideas we normally think about and the functions or ways in which these objects and ideas are normally used, (b) provides supportive cues for everyday problem solving, (c) provides the social situations in which we act and shape our roles, actions, and expectations within these settings, and (d) specifies what an acceptable answer or response is. Consequently, when thinking skills develop in one setting – for example, in the home – specific expectations, rules, and evaluation criteria shape the way those skills are used. When the child enters another context – say, the school – the child's performance may not meet the implicit criteria for good thinking in the new setting because the child is operating from a different set of guidelines. To make this idea more concrete, we now turn to some examples of the influence of contextual factors on children's school performance.

Effect of Context on Children's School Performance

In this section, we present a model of the way factors outside of the school can influence the development of children's thinking skills and children's performance in school (fig. 1). We focus on only one contextual factor – the influence of parents. We believe that, in general, parents are the primary social agents affecting children's early cognitive development.

First, we believe that both home and school are part of the child's greater physical and social environment. The home environment, as characterized by parents' beliefs and attitudes, will match to greater and lesser degrees the beliefs and attitudes of the general population – hence, the home is placed partially within and partially outside of the general environment. If one considers minority cultural groups within the country, one can see similarities and differences in beliefs, compared to dominant cultural groups. In particular, there may be greater and lesser amounts of

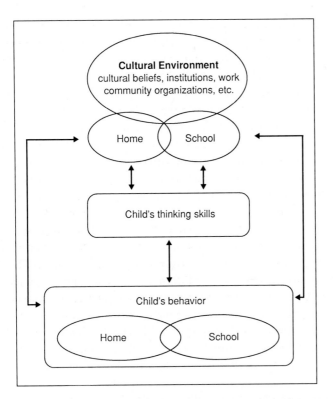

Fig. 1. The interaction of home and school contexts and their influence on children's thinking skills.

overlap between parents' beliefs and attitudes about childrearing, child development, and education and the beliefs and attitudes of the child's teachers in the school setting. In figure 1, we have also placed the school setting partially within and partially outside the general culture. Typically, the beliefs and attitudes of school personnel and the school culture itself are considered to be an important part of the general culture of the country. However, as we argue in the next section, we believe that the school context differs in some very important ways from non-school contexts that are part of the greater environment.

According to our model, both parents' beliefs and behaviors and teachers' beliefs and behaviors affect the development of the child's thinking skills. The overlap in those circles indicates the degree to which parents and teachers have similar beliefs about, for example, expectations for children's behavior, what constitutes intelligent behavior and good problem-solving strategies, expectations for adult-child social roles, and education. If there is a lot of agreement between parents and teachers in what they value and how they believe those behaviors and skills can be developed, then both may encourage the development of the same kinds of thinking skills. If there is very little agreement between parents and teachers, then they may encourage very different thinking skills and problem-solving strategies. That is, the child may develop different rules for thinking and problem solving, some of which are applied at home and some of which are only used at school. In turn, the similarity between the child's behavior at home and at school will depend on the similarity between parents' beliefs and teachers' beliefs. Problems arise when the child carries over implicit rules about thinking and behaving from one setting that do not match the implicit rules that govern the other setting. For example, Heath [1983] described a community in which children are encouraged to generate clever put-downs and sharp verbal retorts in response to teasing from peers and adults. Being able to assess an 'opponent's' weak areas and to come up with a pointed, but funny insult requires verbal ability, flexible thinking, and the ability to deal with novelty. However, such skillfulness is not likely to be appreciated by the teacher who suffers the losing end of a verbal challenge.

To illustrate these ideas more fully, we now focus on how the home environment, as characterized by parental beliefs, can affect the way children deal with school. Several ethnographic studies [Heath, 1983; Mehan, 1979; Ogbu, 1974; Rist, 1973] have described ways in which students from different cultural groups deal with academic and social problems in school settings. These studies suggest that: (a) the match between the values and methods of learning in the school system and the home system vary greatly across subcultural groups in America [Heath, 1983]; (b) success as a student depends in part on understanding the school culture, knowing the implicit rules that govern behavior [Mehan, 1979]; and (c) skills and abilities developed in the home environment can actually work against children in the school environment [Heath, 1983]. The end result is that children are not equally equipped by their home environments for the transition into school – not because intellectual development is not valued in the home setting, but because the particular abilities and styles of teaching used in the home may be very different from the ones that are used in schools. Unfortunately, teachers may misinterpret a child's apparently slow learning as being due to the child's general ability, rather than due to a mismatch between the child's home learning situation and the child's school learning situation. For example, parents may emphasize rote memory of information and gauge children's understanding of things by their ability to recite information verbatim. On the one hand, practice in verbatim recall of knowledge can certainly help children when they study for spelling tests. However, it does not prepare children for the task of explaining ideas in their own words. If a teacher asks a child to express something in his or her own words and the child responds by reciting what the teacher has said, the teacher may assume that the child does not understand the concept very well. However, if the child typically demonstrates what has been learned by reciting what a parent or other adult has taught, the child may, in fact, understand the concept but misunderstand what it means to explain something in your own words.

Sternberg and Suben [1986] have applied the triarchic theory of human intelligence [Sternberg, 1985] to three ethnographic studies as a first step in identifying cognitive processes involved in children's adaptation to school. They matched descriptions of children's behaviors to specific aspects of the triarchic theory to show how cognitive processing may be influenced by early socialization. For example, according to the triarchic theory, a critical metacomponent is allocation of resources. For much of our society, time is one of the resources most carefully apportioned. However, in the Piedmont Carolinas, Heath [1983] studied a community in which very few time limits were placed on tasks and very few activities were actually scheduled. A child in this community may have had literally no experience with being timed in the performance of a cognitive task, prior to school. Hence, to say that one has 30 minutes in which to complete a test may have no functional meaning to the child. Sternberg and Suben suggested that such a child's metacognitive processes may be as well-developed as those of a child from a middle-class home, for example, but the rules that this child uses to make metacognitive decisions (e.g., when given a task to do, the time involved in doing the task is not an important aspect to consider) do not match the implicit rules that govern school settings.

Another basic cognitive process is that of comparing one object or concept to another. Sternberg and Suben discussed the way the process of comparison could be shaped by the home environment. For example, Heath [1983] described a community in which the children seemed to have developed a holistic approach to examining objects – comparing the objects as wholes rather than attribute-by-attribute. Although these children may have been sensitive to shape, color, size, and so on, they did not use these attributes to make judgments as to how two objects might be similar or different. It is not that these children lacked the ability to compare stimuli. Rather, the implicit rules governing object comparisons that had been acquired at home were not the same as the rules assumed by their teachers. Sternberg and Suben argued that the task that children thought they were supposed to be doing was not the 'same' task that the teachers had presented to them. Such misunderstanding can result in poor performance on a task, which unfortunately may be attributed to a lack of ability on the child's part, rather than to an unfamiliarity with the strategies used to accomplish the task.

Even though the ethnographic studies Sternberg and Suben examined were not conducted specifically to study the effects of contextual factors on intellectual development, their analyses identify potential problems in the development of specific cognitive processes that may contribute to poor school performance. Currently, we are conducting a study that examines the relation between parental beliefs and children's early school performance. Kindergarten, first-, and second-grade children (ages 5–7) from schools with very diverse ethnic populations, their parents, and their teachers participated in this project. We are particularly interested in four of the ethnic groups: (a) Cambodians, (b) Caucasians, (c) Hispanics of Mexican descent, and (d) Vietnamese.

Parents completed a questionnaire concerned with their beliefs about: (a) what teachers in first- and second-grade classrooms should do (e.g., teachers should teach children how to ask questions and think about problems); (b) what parents should do with first-grade children (e.g., parents should take children to see new places and do new things); (c) what practical tasks first-grade children should be able to do (e.g., first-grade children should take care of their own belongings); and (d) how effective they think they are as parents (e.g., there are many things I feel I can do to help my child to do well in school). Children were tested at their schools in groups and were given a modified version of the Sternberg Triarchic Abilities Test [Sternberg, in preparation], which has four subscales: (a) componential processing on academic tasks, (b) coping with novelty tasks, (c) practical knowledge and abilities tasks, and (d) automatization tasks. Their teachers rated both academic performance and social behavior of the children.

Our preliminary analyses indicate, first, that there are differences across ethnic groups on the parental-belief scales and that different scales are important for predicting children's test scores across ethnic groups. For example, the majority of the Cambodian parents thought it very important for teachers to do things related to conformity (e.g., teachers should teach children to listen to their teachers and to follow directions). In the other three groups, the majority of parents thought it only somewhat important for teachers to encourage conforming behaviors. In contrast, the majority of parents in all four groups indicated that it is somewhat important or very important for teachers to encourage autonomous thinking and social behavior. Clearly, it is not the case that the Cambodian parents do not value independent, autonomous behavior in their children. Rather, we believe that Cambodian parents may value conforming behavior so highly because learning classroom rules and learning to obey their teachers helps the acculturation of Cambodian children. All of the Cambodian parents in our sample are immigrants. Most have had little formal education either in Cambodia or in the USA. School is a major part of the acculturation process for Cambodian families.

Parents did not differ across ethnic groups with respect to how important they thought it was for children to be able to do various practical tasks – such as having regular chores to do at home. However, within the Cambodian and Vietnamese groups, those parents who thought it more important for children to develop practical knowledge had children with higher total scores on the Triarchic Abilities Test.

Among the Caucasian and the Mexican-American groups, the most important belief scale for predicting children's scores had to do with things parents could do that might inhibit the development of coping-with-novelty skills (e.g., parents should have first graders tell only true stories and be very accurate in what they say; parents should teach first graders to stay inside the lines when they color a picture). Higher ratings on this scale were related to lower children's scores. The Caucasian and Mexican-American parents who believe it is very important for parents to engage in what we might call coping-with-novelty inhibitors still want their children to be intelligent; they simply have different ideas about what parents should do to aid their children's cognitive development.

Thus, we are finding that parents have different ideas about what parents and teachers should do to help children develop and that these beliefs are related to children's cognitive development and to children's school achievement. These data demonstrate that a contextual factor outside of the school setting – namely, parents – can affect the way the children behave at school.

Effect of the School Context on Children's Thinking

We have presented a model of the ways in which one contextual factor external to the classroom – namely, the home – affects the development and teaching of thinking skills within the classroom. In our model, we propose that the school context, although typically thought to be a good representation of the general culture, should be placed partially within and partially outside the general cultural context. In this section, we argue that the school context differs in some important aspects from other settings within the general culture – especially with respect to the application of thinking skills.

The critical feature of the school context that affects the development of thinking skills is the academic framework in which the skills are taught. What do we mean by academic framework? In the last two decades, many psychologists have proposed that people have different sorts of knowledge. One dichotomy is academic versus practical knowledge [Goodnow, 1976, 1984; Neisser, 1976; Rogoff and Lave, 1984; Sternberg and Wagner, 1986]. Neisser's [1976] definition of academic knowledge is knowledge (a) that is not relevant to one's life, (b) that is generally tested in school with sets of rather arbitrary problems that have a single correct solution, and (c) that one has little intrinsic motivation to learn. Academic problems are the kinds of problems that make up standard intelligence tests. Such tests do well to predict school performance, but do poorly in predicting performance on non-school tasks that involve complex cognitive processing, such as racetrack handicapping [Ceci and Liker, 1986] or job performance [Sternberg and Wagner, 1986]. Practical knowledge, on the other hand, is knowledge that is at the heart of one's life. Practical knowledge is information that one uses in everyday situations, in the 'real world' [Rogoff and Lave, 1984].

Are there truly two types of knowledge – academic and practical? If one attempts to apply the definitions of academic and practical knowledge to the many different instances we all know, the distinctions grow fuzzy. Although the categories are useful and one can easily identify the prototypic instances, perhaps there is another way of making this distinction. Perhaps we simply have knowledge that has been contextualized for different purposes.

The distinction between academic and practical knowledge turns on the notion of being 'relevant to the real world'. We learn to use objects, ideas, and procedures for particular purposes. The contextualization that occurs during the acquisition of knowledge seems to make a difference in how we can use that knowledge on subsequent occasions. (See, for example, the Laboratory of Comparative Human Cognition's discussion of functional familiarity [1982].) School is part of the child's real world. Doing problems in school is relevant to the child's life. Perhaps it is not that academic knowledge is irrelevant and unuseful for solving real life problems, but rather that the information and skills that are learned in school are *contextualized so that they only seem relevant for doing the kinds of problems that are found in school.* The school context in which the knowledge is presented and learned does not make that knowledge seem functionally relevant to other situations. Why not?

The basic problem with teaching thinking skills in the school context is that the school context is *not* like the world outside of school in many ways. In school, academic problems are presented to the student. Usually the procedure for solving the problem has just recently been provided to the student, and all of the relevant information needed for solving the problem is given in the problem statement. Oftentimes, there is only one correct solution, and the student can get immediate feedback on his or her answer by asking the teacher or checking in the back of the book. The problems and the problem solving are neat and clean. Life outside of school is not neat and clean. Non-academic problems are messy, ill-defined, and sometimes unanswerable problems. With non-academic problems, even the first step of identifying that there is a problem to solve can separate those who succeed from those who fail. For better and for worse, with non-academic problems, people do not always 'follow the rules'. On the positive side, short-cuts are allowed, and intuitive, innovative procedures that 'work' are applauded, even if they bypass time-honored traditions. One does not have to follow a set procedure for solving the problem and serendipitous solutions, perhaps suggested by the environment, can be employed. On the negative side, the rules we learn in school about cooperating with others, respecting others' feelings and opinions, and compromising to reach mutually acceptable decisions are not always observed by colleagues at work, and group problem solving can be horrendous. The social roles that children have in school limit the amount of responsibility that they have to assume in order to function within the school context. Yes, children have to do their assignments, but the task, the way to do the task, and the evaluation criteria are specified by the teacher. Yes, the children have to get along with other children, but oftentimes when even minor conflicts arise, an adult steps in to arbitrate the situation. A child who simply does what he or she is told can succeed in school. Most of the decisions are made for the child. An adult will flounder through life if he or she is waiting for someone to say which career path to follow, what priorities should be set, what tasks should be done, and what procedures to follow.

Ironically, becoming skillful at academic problem solving does not even guarantee later success in academic professions! Those involved in the training of graduate students know that the analytical skills that enable students to do well on multiple-choice tests, to critique other people's research, to do papers, and even to be admitted to graduate school are not the only skills needed to become a creative, insightful top-quality scientist. Brown et al. [1989] argue, for example, that the way mathematicians use mathematical formulae is different from the way students are taught to use them, or more broadly, that 'school activity' or school use of knowledge is different from 'authentic activity' or knowledge use by practitioners in the domain. Scientists – even those in academic ivory towers – work on messy, ill-defined problems. Furthermore, the successful scientist is the one who not only finds solutions to problems that others have recognized, but also finds problems that others have not yet identified.

Because thinking skills are contextualized, when children develop their thinking skills by working on school problems, they do not necessarily apply these skills to problems outside of school. But, if the school context is the wrong context for teaching thinking skills that will be used in a wide variety of contexts, where should we be teaching thinking skills? Or, what can we do to make the school context a more effective context for teaching thinking skills?

Making School an Effective Context for Teaching Thinking Skills

To say that context affects cognition is to say nothing new. And, to say that context affects cognition is really to say two different things. In this chapter, we have proposed that context affects the development and teaching of thinking skills in two distinct ways: (a) Environmental factors outside the classroom affect the ways in which children are influenced by instruction on thinking skills and their performance on school tasks. (b) School has a contextualizing effect on the development of thinking skills. Hence, the school context may work against the transfer of those thinking skills to situations outside of school. These ideas have definite implications for the development of thinking skills curricula.

School: A Context of Multiple Subject Areas

If thinking skills are learned in context, then a skill learned in one domain will not necessarily transfer automatically to a second domain. Therefore, we believe that skills must be taught in multiple domains. School curricula cross a broad spectrum of content domains, such as literature, mathematics, history, and science. Consequently, schools can teach thinking skills in more than one subject area. Brown et al. [1989] have suggested the metaphor that knowledge can be likened to tools. Tools can be used in different contexts. The techniques for using the same tool in different contexts can be similar or different. Learning to use the tool in different contexts ensures that the tool will be viewed as relevant in multiple contexts, gives the child a richer concept of that tool and its uses, and makes it more likely that the child will later see the tool as being relevant in a new domain. Perkins and Salomon [1989] have proposed that to obtain transfer one either must provide a lot of practice in many different situations or must have students abstract or look for the general principles from specific situations themselves and then encourage students to apply the principles in new and varied situations.

One alternative to teaching thinking skills in multiple content areas is to try to teach them as abstract rules that are not bound to any particular content area. As others have suggested [Adams, 1989; Perkins and Salomon, 1989], we believe that to teach thinking skills as conceptual knowledge, or sets of abstract rules to follow, is probably not to teach thinking skills that will be used by the child in everyday practice. Moreover, so-called 'context-free' examples (such as making inferences about geometric figures) actually do constitute a content domain in which the skills are embedded [Adams, 1989]. Therefore, thinking skills need to be taught and practiced within content domains.

School: A Context with Messy Problems to Identify and to Solve

In order to enable students to use thinking skills in everyday situations, we need to make the school context more like the contexts the child encounters outside of school. We must embed the skills in a context that makes the skills relevant to non-school problems. Our goal in teaching thinking skills is *not* to produce students who can identify and describe a set of thinking skills. Our goal is to produce students who regularly apply thinking skills to all kinds of problems. Therefore, we have to give students problems that are more like non-school problems – problems that are (a) ill-defined, (b) require students to search for relevant information,

(c) allow students to develop 'their own solution paths' [Brown et al., 1989], and (d) allow them to develop the evaluation criteria for the solution. (We are not suggesting that students be allowed to grade all of their projects, merely that students need to have some opportunities to evaluate for themselves whether or not a potential solution is a good one.) Moreover, we must give students opportunities to recognize and find problems to solve on their own.

School: A Context Sensitive to External Influences

In this chapter, we have presented only a few examples of the ways in which one factor – parental beliefs – can affect children's thinking. The potential number of environmental factors that could affect children's thinking are too numerous to consider. What, then, should our first steps be in order to be sensitive to these influences?

First, we need to find out what ideas, beliefs, and implicit rules children already have about good problem solving and good thinking. We cannot assume that their ideas or their parents' beliefs match their teachers' ideas. Second, we need to be explicit about the applications of and the evaluation criteria for thinking skills. We cannot assume that children understand the problems and the tasks in the same way that their teachers do. Third, we need to make explicit the implicit rules that govern teacher-student roles and social behavior in the school learning context.

Finally, as we come to a better knowledge and appreciation of the beliefs and rules that guide 'good thinking' for different subcultures within our country, we should be able to identify the situations in which the different sets of 'good thinking rules' can best be applied. Recall Heath's example of children using a holistic approach to compare objects rather than a more analytic, feature-by-feature approach. There are times when switching to a holistic approach can provide new insights into a problem and lead to solution. Our goal in teaching thinking skills should not be a complete replacement of one set of rules for good thinking with another set. Rather, we should take advantage of the diversity in our school settings to stretch our concepts of good thinking.

Acknowledgements

Preparation of this chapter was supported in part by a grant to the authors from the Spencer Foundation. We would like to thank Peter Frensch for his comments on earlier versions of the manuscript.

References

Adams, M.J. (1989). Thinking skills curricula: Their promise and progress. *Educational Psychologist, 24,* 25–77.

Brown, J.S., Collins, A., & Duguid, P. (1989). Situated cognition and the culture of learning. *Educational Researcher, 18,* 32–42.

Bronfenbrenner, U. (1977). Toward an experimental ecology of human development. *American Psychologist, 32,* 513–531.

Bronfenbrenner, U. (1979). *The ecology of human development.* Cambridge MA: Harvard University Press.

Ceci, S.J., & Liker, J. (1986). Academic and nonacademic intelligence: an experimental separation. In R.J. Sternberg (Ed.), *Practical intelligence: Nature and origins of competence in the everyday world* (pp. 119–142). New York: Cambridge University Press.

Cole, M., Gay, J., Glick, J., & Sharp, D. (1971). *The cultural context of learning and thinking.* New York: Basic Books.

Gelman, R. (1978). Cognitive development. *Annual Review of Psychology, 29,* 297–332.

Goodnow, J.J. (1976). The nature of intelligent behavior: Questions raised by cross-cultural studies. In L.B. Resnick (Ed.), *The nature of intelligence* (pp. 169–188). Hillsdale NJ: Erlbaum.

Goodnow, J.J. (1984). On being judged intelligent. *International Journal of Psychology, 19,* 391–406.

Heath, S.B. (1983). *Ways with words.* New York: Cambridge University Press.

Laboratory of Comparative Human Cognition (1982). Culture and intelligence. In R. J. Sternberg (Ed.), *Handbook of Human Intelligence* (pp. 642–719). New York: Cambridge University Press.

Lantz, D. (1979). A cross-cultural comparison of communication abilities. Some effects of age, schooling and culture. *International Journal of Psychology, 14,* 171–183.

Luria, A.R. (1976). *Cognitive development: Its cultural and social foundations.* (Translated by M. Lopez-Morillas & L. Solotaroff. Edited by M. Cole.) Cambridge MA: Harvard University Press.

Mehan, H. (1979). *Learning lessons: Social organization in the classroom.* Cambridge MA: Harvard University Press.

Neisser, U. (1976). *Cognition and reality.* San Francisco: Freeman.

Ogbu, J. (1974). *The next generation: An ethnography of education in an urban neighborhood.* New York: Academic Press.

Okagaki, L., & Sternberg R.J. (in preparation). Parents' beliefs about education, intelligence, and parenting.

Perkins, D.N., & Salomon, G. (1989). Are cognitive skills context-bound? *Educational Researcher, 18,* 16–25.

Rist, R. (1973). *The urban school: A factory for failure.* Cambridge MA: MIT Press.

Rogoff, B. (1982). Integrating context and cognitive development. In M.E. Lamb & A.L. Brown (Eds.), *Advances in developmental psychology* (Vol. 2, pp. 125–170). Hillsdale NJ: Erlbaum.

Rogoff, B., & Lave, J. (Eds.). (1984). *Everyday cognition.* Cambridge MA: Harvard University Press.

Scribner, S. (1984). Studying working intelligence. In B. Rogoff & J. Lave (Eds.), *Everyday cognition*. Cambridge MA: Harvard University Press.

Scribner, S. (1986). Thinking in action: some characteristics of practical thought. In R.J. Sternberg & R.K. Wagner (Eds.), *Practical intelligence: Nature and origins of competence in the everyday world* (pp. 13–30). New York: Cambridge University Press.

Sternberg, R.J. (1985). *Beyond IQ: A triarchic theory of human intelligence.* New York: Cambridge University Press.

Sternberg, R.J. (in press). *Sternberg Triarchic Abilities Test.* San Antonio TX: The Psychological Corporation.

Sternberg, R.J., & Suben, J.G. (1986). The socialization of intelligence. In M. Perlmutter (Ed.), Perspectives on intellectual development. *Minnesota symposia on child psychology* (Vol. 19, pp. 201–235). Hillsdale NJ. Erlbaum.

Sternberg, R.J., & Wagner, R.K. (Eds.) (1986). *Practical intelligence: Nature and origins of competence in the everyday world.* New York: Cambridge University Press.

Kuhn D (ed): Developmental Perspectives on Teaching and Learning Thinking Skills.
Contrib Hum Dev. Basel, Karger, 1990, vol 21, pp 79–94

Approaching School Intelligently: An Infusion Approach

Mara Krechevsky, Howard Gardner

Educational interventions grounded in theory exhibit a distinctly different flavor from those which grow out of practice. Consider, for example, the difference between Boole's *Laws of thought* [1854] and Edwards' *Drawing on the right side of the brain* [1979]. Boole's volume was designed to help people think; yet, it reflects the aesthetics of the logician rather than the kinds of practical problems that the ordinary rational (or irrational) person must confront in daily life. Edwards' book offers a promissory note that one may invoke a typically underutilized set of brain structures in becoming a better artist. But the appeal of the book inheres in its set of exercises, which are quite effective in helping nascent drawers observe and depict their subjects in a representationally faithful fashion.

The distance between a textbook on human memory and the 'method of Simonides' may seem slimmer, but the difference in accent is parallel. The theorist whose work is summarized in the text is trying to flesh out the basic laws of memory. These principles should explain the slavish recall of nonsense syllables as well as reconstruction of the gist of a story. Simonides, in contrast, wanted simply a method that could help him to recall the identities of a large number of guests gathered around a table at a fateful dinner.

Reverberations of these tensions are found today in the flood of materials being devised to improve thinking skills. On the one hand, nearly every psychologist or 'cognitive scientist' who has ever uttered the word 'thinking' has at least asked him- or herself whether he or she might have something useful to contribute to the current intellectual malaise in American schools. On the other hand, a large number of current teachers, former teachers, and other 'practitioners' have drawn on *their* lore. They too hope to popularize methods that will improve the thinking processes and/or the thought-filled products of school children. While each of these 'interest groups' is comfortably rooted in its own history, there is a certain hankering for the other perspective. Scientific theorists wish that their methods could be instantly transferred to the untidy and unpredictable classroom, while practitioners search for the generative power of an appropriate theoretical base for their techniques.

Like the other authors represented in this volume, we are clearly part of the research community and presumably suffer from the same limitations of experience and perspective. The particular slant that we have taken on issues of thinking grows out of the theory of multiple intelligences, on which Gardner and his associates have been working for the last decade. Yet, it is a cardinal principle of this theory that thinking does not and cannot occur apart from interaction with real materials in a living context. At the same time, we would argue, an approach to thinking that aspires to have an effect in the schools must reflect the perceived needs of the students for help in various scholastic tasks and the reality of conditions inside ordinary schools, where 25 or 30 students inhabit the same room with the same teacher for several hours a day. In what follows, as we put forth the theoretical rationale for our approach to thinking, we seek to bear in mind these important contextual factors.

A New Conception of Intelligence

Traditionally, intelligence has been considered a general ability found in varying degrees in all individuals and especially critical for successful performance in school. Since the time of Plato, this unitary view of the mind has been a dominant influence in Western thought. In recent years, however, an alternative view has been put forth which suggests that the mind is organized into relatively independent realms of functioning [Feldman, 1980, 1986; Fodor, 1983; Gardner, 1983]. The theory of multiple intelligences (hereafter, MI theory), discussed in detail in *Frames of mind* [Gardner, 1983], represents one such pluralistic approach to the notion of intelligence. In MI theory, intelligence is defined as the ability to solve problems or fashion products that are valued in one or more cultural settings. Gardner proposes that all normal individuals are capable of at least seven relatively autonomous forms of intellectual accomplishment: linguistic, musical, logical-mathematical, spatial, bodily-kinesthetic, interpersonal and intrapersonal.

In his efforts to identify and conceptualize a candidate intelligence, Gardner surveyed a wide range of sources: research on the developmental trajectories of different capacities in normal and gifted individuals; the breakdown of these capacities under conditions of brain damage; studies of exceptional populations exhibiting highly jagged profiles (e.g., 'idiot savants', prodigies, and autistic children); a plausible evolutionary history; psychometric findings; studies of transfer and generalization of skills; and cross-cultural accounts of cognition. Each intelligence has one or more core information-processing operations or mechanisms that enable individuals to make sense of specific kinds of input. For example, core operations of musical intelligence include sensitivity to pitch, rhythm, and timbre, while the capacity to represent and manipulate spatial configurations is a core operation of spatial intelligence. An intelligence must also be susceptible to encoding in a symbol system – a culturally contrived system of meaning that captures and transmits knowledge, such as spoken language or pictorial systems.

Intelligences are always negotiated within the context of the current array of fields and disciplines represented in the schools and society at large. Although based initially on a biological potential, intelligences are inevitably expressed as a result of intersecting genetic and environmental factors. They do not ordinarily function in isolation, except in certain exceptional populations, such as 'idiot savants'. Each culture emphasizes a different set of intelligences and combination of intelligences. These intelligences are embedded (or perhaps embodied) in the employment of the various symbol systems, notational systems, e.g., musical or mathematical notation, and fields of knowledge, e.g., graphic design or nuclear physics [Csikszentmihalyi and Robinson, 1986].

In most Western cultures, the task of learning the notational systems is carried out in the relatively decontextualized setting of schools. Many students cannot connect their more commonsense knowledge to cognate concepts presented in a school context. To take one well-known example, when a group of students was presented the problem of how many buses would be required to transport 1,128 soldiers if each bus held 36 soldiers, most replied '31, remainder 12'. These students correctly applied the appropriate arithmetic operation, but without regard for the meaning of their answer [Schoenfeld, 1988; Strauss, 1982].

Although school knowledge is often dissociated from real-world contexts, it is in rich, situation-specific contexts that intelligences are typically and productively deployed. The kind of knowledge required in workplaces and in one's personal life usually involves collaborative, contextualized, and situation-specific thinking [Gardner, 1990a; Resnick, 1987; Rogoff and Lave, 1984]. Schools do provide some group activities, but students are usually judged on their individual work. By contrast, in many social and occupational settings, one's ability to communicate effectively and work productively with others is critical to a successful outcome. Furthermore, whereas school learning often features the manipulation of abstract symbols and the execution of 'pure thought' activities, most of the thinking required outside of school is tied to a specific task or goal, whether it be running a business, calculating a batting average, or planning a vacation. In these situations, intrapersonal intelligence – or the ability to recognize which skills are required, and to capitalize on one's strengths and compensate for one's limitations – may be especially important.

Of course, the institution of school itself is a complex one for children to negotiate. School features its own disciplines, codes, notations, and expectations which, for better or worse, are critical to survival in the West. Children who find it difficult to 'decode' school are likely to be at risk for future problems, in or outside of school. While a great deal of research has focused on the 'academic' intelligences of language and logic and on the other main academic disciplines, less effort has been devoted to what it takes to survive and thrive in the environment of school more generally. Because school plays such a central role in our culture, it is important to examine those intelligences and skills needed for students to survive and flourish in the system.

The Practical Intelligence for School (PIFS) Project

As one turns one's attention to a specific setting like school, the question arises of how best to aid students in adjusting to and mastering that environment. In our view, a comprehensive effort to enhance a student's 'school intelligences' must address at least several factors. For example, such an effort has to address conditions particular to that environment, ranging from the physical set-up of classes to the demands of particular disciplines. It also has to consider the particular skills that students initially bring to the tasks and the general environment of school, as well as the optimal pedagogical means for helping students to enhance or alter their current skills and attitudes, so that they are more appropriate for the demands of the school context. Finally, the production of a set of measures that can indicate the way in which a prescribed intervention achieves (or fails to achieve) its effect is also needed. In all probability, no single current theoretical framework is adequate to incorporate all of these factors, though important components of such an account can be found in the works of Bruner et al. [1966], Scribner and Cole [1973], and Wagner and Stevenson [1982].

Two recent approaches have a dual concern with the development of intelligence in general and practical survival in specific contexts such as school. The first, Sternberg's [1985, 1988] triarchic theory of intelligence, defines intelligence in terms of (1) the internal world of the individual (the information-processing components of metacognitive, performance and knowledge-acquisition components); (2) the external world of the individual (the individual's ability to adapt to and shape existing environments, or select new ones); and (3) the experience of the individual in the world (how the individual copes with novelty and automatizes information processing). As already noted, the second approach – Gardner's MI theory – stresses the importance of skills being used in specific cultural contexts. In addition, particular intelligences are keyed to particular school subject matters, e.g., English and history stress linguistic intelligence, whereas math and science draw on logical-mathematical intelligence. Adaptation to the social environment of school calls upon interpersonal intelligence, while having a sense of oneself as a learner, with particular strengths, weaknesses, and stylistic features, draws upon intrapersonal intelligence.

In recently launched collaborative research, Gardner, Sternberg, and their colleagues are seeking to identify how best to prepare students 'at risk for school failure' for successful performance in school and subsequent institutional and occupational settings. The project was designed to develop and test a multifaceted model of *practical intelligence for school* (PIFS), drawing on both the MI and the triarchic theories of intelligence. In particular, it seemed important to determine how the academic intelligences work together with the more practical inter- and intrapersonal intelligences to produce a successful scholastic experience. We also wanted to examine the relationship of academic success to the functions of adaptation to, selection of, and shaping of environments, outlined in Sternberg's 'contextual subtheory'. Our underlying premise was that students who thrive in school need to learn, apply, and integrate both academic knowledge about subject domains and practical knowledge about themselves, academic tasks, and the school system at large.

As we formulated it, PIFS requires knowledge in three broad areas: (1) one's own intellectual profile, learning styles and strategies; (2) the structure and learning of academic tasks; and (3) the school as a complex social system. These categories can also be articulated in MI terms: The first represents intrapersonal intelligence. The second represents the manifestation of academic intelligences and combinations of intelligences in particular domains. (For example, science involves logical-mathematical competence more than linguistic ability, and some spatial ability; social studies draws upon its own blend of linguistic and logical competences.) The third category reflects primarily interpersonal intelligence.

The PIFS intervention efforts target the middle-school population for a number of reasons. The sixth and seventh grades (ages 11–12), in particular, are a time when students should have already developed considerable practical knowledge about the school environment, and a time after which lack of such knowledge proves increasingly deleterious to scholastic performance. Youths in early adolescence are starting to undergo major physical, intellectual, and emotional growth and change. They are becoming increasingly independent, which is reflected in the activities and projects they will be asked to carry out. Thus, the middle-school years represent an important transition between the elementary grades and high school.

In light of these concerns, we embarked on a multi-pronged attack on the issue of practical intelligences. Our approach involved identification of students' own knowledge about the topic, determining students' and teachers' understanding of the sources and nature of the trouble spots, designing rich and inviting curricula to address the problem areas directly and imaginatively, piloting and implementing PIFS curricular units in a number of settings, and devising appropriate evaluation schemes.

The PIFS Interviews

As indicated, we wanted to determine what the students themselves understood about their roles as students. Thus, we conducted a series of in-depth interviews with 50 fifth and sixth graders (10–11 years old) from a variety of socioeconomic backgrounds in five schools in the Boston area. The interviews elicited student views on such topics as study habits, the evaluation process, subject matter differences, the demands of academic tasks, the roles of teachers and administrators, peer interactions, and the nature of the school system. After transcribing and analyzing the responses, we outlined a hierarchical taxonomy of PIFS profiles, dividing students into categories based on whether they exhibited characteristics of a 'high', 'middle', or 'low' PIFS profile. Our major findings are summarized here. (For a full report, see Goldman et al. [1988].)

We focus here on the three main factors that differentiated low from high PIFS profile students – elaboration of responses, awareness of strategies and resources, and sense of self as learner. However, an important similarity emerged in the limited understanding exhibited by both high and low PIFS students regarding similarities and differences among different subject matters. These factors had direct implications for the infusion approach and were incorporated into the themes and guiding principles for the curriculum.

Elaboration of Responses. Low profile students seemed restricted by the limited vocabulary which they could draw on for discussion of the PIFS issues. They found it difficult to explain why they found certain subjects hard or easy or why they preferred one subject to another. High profile students were more likely to offer reasons spontaneously for their answers and were better able to differentiate among courses, academic tasks, and personal strengths and weaknesses. However, 'verbal molecules' [Strauss, 1988], or truisms, were common among both low and high profile students, e.g., 'A good student is one who pays attention' or 'Anyone can do better if she tries'. In fact, the majority of students could be considered 'incremental' rather than 'entity' theorists [Dweck and Elliott, 1983], at least at the rhetorical level. Incremental theorists view intelligence as a set of skills that can be improved through effort, whereas entity theorists consider intelligence to be more global and stable. Yet, although both lows and highs espoused an incrementalist view in their responses, few lows were able to articulate more specifically how academic performance might be improved. Finally, fifth graders seemed significantly more literal than sixth graders in their thinking ('A bad teacher is one who is absent a lot'; 'A bad textbook is one with a page ripped out'; 'A good school is not dirty'); this result helped to motivate our decision to focus on the latter grade.

Strategies and Resources. Highs and lows also varied greatly in their awareness and use of strategies for studying, as well as their resourcefulness in seeking help. Highs understood their strengths and weaknesses and varied their approaches to different subjects accordingly. They were also able to call upon teachers, friends, parents and older siblings for encouragement, critique, instruction, and motivation. Lows, in contrast, advocated a more global, all-encompassing strategy: 'Try harder and study more'. As one boy explained, 'Everything helps a little, but not that much'. When asked what his 'resource period' was, he said, 'I don't know, I never asked'. His responses suggested helplessness, passivity, and magical thinking. School was a mystery to him.

Self as Learner. Finally, highs evinced a strong sense of themselves as learners. They related their various school tasks to both long-term and personal goals. Lows often espoused a 'disciplinarian' viewpoint: 'You do homework because you have to'; 'A good test is a hard one'; 'A good teacher is a strict one'. 'Good' means 'hard', and 'learning' means 'suffering'. While most lows seemed to have a limited or negative identity as learners, they usually revealed at least one area in which they could make appropriate discriminations and value judgments. For example, one student, in discussing team sports, was able to articulate the qualities of a good coach, the connections between practice and performance, the nature of his time commitments, and so forth. Such topics, ranging from dancing and designing to athletics and auto mechanics, represented areas in which students were both interested and, usually, in which they felt capable. These potential 'hooks' might be used to exploit student interest and confidence in one domain of knowledge as a means to facilitate growth in other domains.

Subject Matter Differences. An unexpected similarity between highs and lows was the limited understanding they displayed of the kinds of skills and underlying reasoning processes entailed in different subject matters. In fact, without explicit training, youngsters at this age appear oblivious to cross-disciplinary similarities and differences. Most students defined subjects in terms of content:

> In science you learn about nature; in English, they are teaching about how to talk properly – like 'I learned about frogs today, ain't that nice' – that's not good English, but it's okay to say in science.

Moreover, students could articulate little, if any, understanding or appreciation of the differing status of knowledge within and across content areas. Many considered facts more important than fiction; textbooks were 'real', and stories were 'fake' and 'just for fun'. One high PIFS student, however, articulated the difference as follows:

Stories ... take you into a different world – and you're off fighting dragons and being in love. And textbooks, you're right down, in earth, this time, this place, doing math ...

Through our interviews, we identified the following themes that permeate each of the PIFS curriculum units: ability and willingness to take an active role as learner; understanding of the learning process involved in different academic activities; and ability to take a pluralistic view of school tasks and roles.

The Infusion Curriculum

In accordance with the theoretical models discussed earlier, we decided to foster PIFS skills via two sets of curriculum modules, one following an 'infusion' and the other a 'separate course' approach. Both infusion and separate-course approaches to teaching thinking have merit. While all domains require some domain-specific skills, there are also more general strategies or heuristics that can be applied across content areas. However, the key issue in determining the value of a thinking skills approach is the *transfer* of knowledge and skills. General skills learned in a separate course are worthwhile only if they prove useful for problem solving in specific subject matter; infusion approaches should be able to demonstrate that the skills learned have some application beyond a specific content area [Nisbet, 1989].

Both sets of PIFS modules were designed to help students to think critically about themselves, academic tasks, and the school environment. The separate-course approach, based on Sternberg's theoretical model, offers a stand-alone curriculum addressing such issues as time management, communication skills, and following directions. On the basis of our own theory, we at Harvard Project Zero elected to use the infusion approach primarily, although we hope ultimately to combine the two approaches. Here we focus on the infusion approach.

The aim of the PIFS infusion curriculum is to promote transfer by explicitly directing students' attention to how problems in different domains relate to each other and by providing students with the tools and techniques for self-monitoring in different subject matters. The approach is based on two fundamental assumptions of MI theory: (1) one learns information best when it is presented in a rich context; and (2) it is difficult to secure transfer from separate courses or isolated definitions and skills to the kinds of problems that arise unexpectedly in the course of school work or life [Brown and Campione, 1984; Perkins and Salomon, 1989].

The infusion approach can be thought of as a 'meta-curriculum' that serves as a bridge between standard curricula (math word problems, geography, vocabulary, etc.) and a decontextualized thinking or study-skills curriculum that purports to be applicable across subject matter. The curriculum consists of a set of infusion units intended to help students better understand the reasons for the types of tasks they are assigned in school, and how best to accomplish them. The units try to foster a self-monitoring and a self-reflectiveness directly related to the nature and problems of the specific content area in which a student is working [Hyde and Bizar, 1989]. This self-understanding, a constituent of intrapersonal intelligence, is directly related to the themes noted above. In particular, the units build on those areas identified by both students and teachers as difficult for students, e.g., the process of revision, and organizing and presenting one's work.

The 16 infusion units currently cover topics in social studies, mathematics, reading and writing, and more general topics such as organizing and presenting work and taking tests, that draw on specific subject matter instantiations. Two examples of units follow.

'Choosing a Project'. The objective of this unit is to help students choose and plan school projects more effectively. Projects represent a rich alternative to worksheets, comprehension questions, and standardized tests. They provide students with the opportunity to study a topic in depth, to raise questions and explore answers, and to determine the best form for demonstrating newly acquired expertise. However, while students are often absorbed in a variety of extracurricular projects such as writing rap songs and building skateboard ramps, they are often less engaged in executing school projects. Many find it difficult to get started; or they may choose topics that are either too narrow or too broad, or topics in which they exhibit scant interest.

The 'Choosing a Project' unit includes three sets of activities: 'Understanding Projects', 'Choosing a Project Appropriate to You', and 'Planning a Project Appropriate to the Audience and Resources'. The first set of activities encourages students to examine the similarities and differences between personal and school projects and between school projects and other school assignments. They also address the definition, goals, and criteria for success of various projects. The remaining activities encourage students to use their past experiences with projects to plan new projects that (1) relate to their abilities, interests, and relative expertise, and (2) can be carried out within the constraints of the assignment.

'Finding the Right Mathematical Tools'. The goal of this unit is to familiarize students with a range of mathematical resources and to help students apply resources appropriate to particular problem types. Part I invites students to consider the resources with which they are already familiar in their daily life: books, television, recipes, maps, etc. The second part of the unit introduces resources specific to math: calculators, textbooks, measuring tools, tables and charts, etc. The advantages and shortcomings of different

types of resources are identified and discussed through a variety of classroom activities. Focus is on choosing the appropriate resource for a problem type, rather than on generating the final solution. In the last section, students reflect on their own patterns of error as well as their skills in using the various resources.

PIFS Infusion Principles

Each PIFS infusion unit reflects some of the following principles.

Practical intelligence skills are most fruitfully nurtured in domain-specific contexts. The topics addressed by the PIFS units are always explored in the context of the subject matter; thus, the types of resources that are important for mathematics are considered separately from those useful for social studies. These differences are further highlighted and contrasted in order to sensitize students to the nature of various subject matters. In the 'Mathematical Tools' unit, students study the general characteristics, relevance, and reliability of the different types of mathematical resources for specific categories of math problems. In a 'Reliability of Sources' unit, students examine potential causes of unreliability specific to the domain of social studies – lack of corroboration or expertise, observer bias, perceptual inaccuracy, and so forth.

Concepts that present difficulties for students should be analyzed and clarified in focused activities. Each problem area is analyzed in order to identify specific sources of difficulty, which are then addressed in manageable chunks via short exercises. The problems are worked through in the context of an actual assignment, rather than in isolation. In the 'Choosing a Project' unit, such identified trouble spots as choice of topic, planning within the constraints of time and resources, monitoring one's progress, and responding to feedback are each considered in turn. A 'Notetaking' unit includes brief exercises intended to let students know that taking notes can be quickly and easily accomplished. A note can be as simple as a single 'key word' that triggers other information. Students begin by identifying key words in single sentences, moving on to longer pieces of text. Of course, establishing the right kind of classroom atmosphere and providing appropriate follow-up activities are also important to ensure that the benefits of the core activities are reinforced.

Concepts taught in the PIFS units are most effectively implemented when used in service of a particular purpose. The units highlight and exemplify the fact that most tasks, projects, assignments, indeed most work, are undertaken for a particular purpose. In the 'Mathematical Tools' unit, students compare the purpose of resources used in their personal lives and in math class. They are also asked to write problems for which particular resources would be appropriate. One of the goals of the unit is to increase students' independence and resourcefulness by explicitly linking different math resources to situations in which students typically have difficulties. In a geography unit, students engage in a number of activities that illustrate that maps are always drawn for a specific purpose, with a particular audience in mind.

Students acquire knowledge best when it is related to their own sets of abilities and interests. Each PIFS unit is individualized in order to: (1) enrich assignments by bringing in students' own interests from their scholastic or nonscholastic experience; (2) draw on students' strengths by reflecting their unique sets of intelligences; and (3) connect students' prior projects and work (old papers or tests, habitual sources or patterns of error, etc.) to current assignments. As already noted, the 'Projects' unit addresses each of the above points. The 'Discovering Your Learning Profile' unit is comprised of activities that explicitly encourage students to contemplate their various 'intelligences' and learning styles. If a student recognizes that she has limited linguistic intelligence, she may need to put extra effort into studying for a vocabulary test. If she is aware of her strong spatial intelligence, she may be able to study vocabulary more effectively by memorizing words and their definitions in terms of their location on a study sheet or translating definitions into concrete images.

Practical intelligence skills are most powerfully integrated when presented in both scholastic and real-world contexts. The PIFS skills addressed by the units are situated in both academic and real-world settings to help students establish connections to their own experience. For example, students consider how mathematical resources are useful not just for their homework assignments, but when planning a trip, baking cookies, or justifying an increase in one's allowance. The 'Notetaking' unit identifies situations in which notetaking occurs, perhaps without students recognizing it as such, e.g., phone messages and shopping lists. The 'Why Go To School' unit encourages thought about the function of school, its effect on quality of life, alternative methods of education, and the reality and myths (often fostered by television portrayals) of the working world. Metaphors and analogies are also used where helpful to demystify difficult concepts and facilitate understanding. These metaphors help make a concept like revision more accessible and memorable by tying it to an image students can readily recognize and understand, such as movie-making, sports practice, or choosing an outfit. Trying to solve math problems without the right resources is compared to a mechanic trying to get the job done without a box of tools.

Students benefit from a focus on process as well as product. While final products and correct answers are clearly important, practical intelligence involves knowing what to do when one gets stuck and how to seek appropriate help. Therefore, the PIFS units often emphasize the process of carrying out an assignment or solving a problem, with reduced emphasis on the actual solution. As mentioned earlier, the 'Mathematical Tools' unit contains many exercises that do not require completion. Rather, students are asked to identify the mathematical resources appropriate for different problems. In the 'Understanding Fiction' unit, students focus on pinpointing the source of their misunderstanding in a work of fiction so that they will be able to ask more precise questions and identify areas requiring further help.

Self-monitoring helps students to take active responsibility for their own learning. Self-monitoring is explicitly encouraged in all of the units before, during, and after the activities. It is not enough simply to learn the skills of practical intelligence; students must also practice overseeing and monitoring their use so that reliance on the teacher is reduced. In mathematics, both the advantages and disadvantages of particular resources are highlighted in an effort to encourage students to think more critically and reflectively about when and how to use different mathematical tools. In the 'Projects' unit, projects undertaken both in and outside of school are examined, compared and evaluated. Students are asked to compare reports written in areas about which they know a great deal to reports written in areas where they have little or no knowledge. As a general rule, students are provided with exemplars illustrating successful and unsuccessful performances in order to provoke more evaluative thinking.

Evaluation of PIFS Units

Practical intelligence skills can be most effectively evaluated by a focus on metacognitive issues as well as on actual task performance. The PIFS evaluation measures assess students' ability-in-context. The measures fall into three categories – definitional, task-oriented, and meta-task. The definitional component addresses students' understanding of the problem, e.g., do they understand the issues addressed by the PIFS unit and why they are important? Such understanding might be exhibited even without mastery of the skills needed to execute the task effectively. The task component samples the actual skills targeted in the units – students may be asked either to start or to complete a task, or perhaps to work through a problem area. Finally, the meta-task component requires students to reflect on the nature of the process or skills involved in a particular task. They are asked to evaluate whether their performances were successful, and if not, how they could be revised or improved.

The following evaluation measures provide examples from the two sample units described earlier. A definitional measure for 'Choosing a Project' asks students to list the factors that should be considered when choosing a particular project. In the 'Mathematical Tools' unit, students are asked to identify situations in which particular math resources would be helpful. The task measure for the 'Projects' unit asks students to complete a planning sheet for a hypothetical project. An equivalent measure for the 'Mathematical Tools' unit gives students a problem, while restricting their access to certain resources, and asks them to generate other options for solving the problem. Finally, one of the meta-task measures for 'Choosing a Project' asks students to critique three completed planning sheets and to make suggestions for improving one of the less promising proposals. In the math unit, students are presented with a scenario in which a hypothetical classmate has used several resources to solve a particularly thorny math problem. They are asked to evaluate the appropriateness of the classmate's work.

The PIFS measures incorporate some of the characteristics of Wiggins' [1989] criteria for 'authentic' tests in that the assessments are contextualized. They reflect realistic complexity; content is mastered as a means, not an end; and students are asked to pose and clarify problems, not just to provide solutions. The evaluation measures are intended to be useful not only as assessment of what the students learned in the PIFS unit, but also as examples of good pedagogy [Gardner, 1990b].

Conclusions

We have described a new curricular approach, designed to aid students in managing the complex and sometimes conflicting demands of school. The overall PIFS approach identifies three major areas of focus for a 'practical intelligence' curriculum and several of the factors critical to such an effort. The PIFS infusion approach reflects, in addition, a number of principles related to the development of an infusion curriculum. It is too early to indicate whether this approach succeeds in its avowed goals, though we can state that the several master teachers who have piloted portions of the curriculum find it congenial to their classroom procedures and goals.

Our treatment raises a number of questions to which we can here provide brief answers. A first question is whether a multiple-intelligences approach can be productive, given the schools' perennial focus on linguistic and logical thinking. It seems clear that certain combinations of intelligences (e.g., linguistic, logical, and certain aspects of interpersonal) are highly prized and rewarded in the scholastic context. It is certainly neither straightforward (nor necessarily desirable) to elevate some of the 'fringe' intelligences to the status of the academic competencies, nor to use them as vehicles of instruction in the standard subject areas. However, students experiencing difficulty in the traditional academic areas seem both to perform better and to feel more empowered when given the chance to exhibit their knowledge and understanding through other than linguistic means.

A second question is whether our own theories have been affected by involvement in this project. We believe that they have in at least two ways. First, MI theory stands to benefit from increased attention to the metacognitive aspects of the several intelligences, just as the metacomponents of the triarchic theory are nuanced by application to different domains. Second, like most psychological theories, our accounts of intelligence have been centered on the cognition of the solitary individual. But once one begins to work in the classroom, it becomes evident that one must confront issues of how students work together on projects as well as how assessment and instruction can work most effectively in the context of such a large group of individuals.

A third question is how the PIFS approach might work if it sought to utilize the infusion and stand-alone curricula to the fullest. We believe that PIFS concepts should be introduced at the beginning of the year, both explicitly and implicitly, with the concepts functioning as 'leitmotifs' in later assignments. Teacher modeling, hands-on activities, and small group work are integral to a PIFS-infused environment, and are recommended in the units [Palincsar and Brown, 1984; Brown and Campione, this volume], as are additional practice and follow-up activities. Our hope is that teachers return to the PIFS units as needed to supplement the existing subject matter curricula, that students learn to call upon the techniques during times of difficulty, and, finally, that students gradually internalize the PIFS techniques and concepts so that they become a standard and readily available part of every child's repertoire.

Finally, the question arises regarding the extent to which the curriculum might be manipulative in spirit or in operation. Although one of the goals of the PIFS curriculum is to help students in their coursework and assignments, there is a fine line between learning to 'psyche out' what teachers want and acquiring the tools to learn on one's own and want to learn more. One criterion of success of the PIFS project is improvement in scholastic performance and student engagement in school. But an even more attractive goal is for students to take responsibility for their own education, even after school is over, so that practical intelligence for schooling becomes practical intelligence for the acquisition of knowledge and understanding throughout life. By expanding the focus of current educational interventions to include practical as well as academic skills, we hope not only to serve a young contemporary Simonides or Boole well, but to help many struggling students become active, planful, and reflective learners.

Acknowledgements

The work described in this chapter was supported by a grant from the James S. McDonnell Foundation. We are grateful to Tina Blythe and Noel White, who gave many helpful comments on earlier drafts.

References

Boole, G. (1984/1952). *The laws of thought.* Lasalle: The Open Court Publishing Co.
Brown, A.L., & Campione, J.C. (1984). Three faces of transfer: Implications for early competence, individual differences, and instruction. In M. Lamb, A. Brown, & B. Rogoff (Eds.), *Advances in developmental psychology* (Vol. 3). Hillsdale: Erlbaum.
Bruner, J., Olver, R., & Greenfield, P. (1966). *Studies in cognitive growth.* New York: Wiley.

Csikszentmihalyi, M., & Robinson, R. (1986). Culture, time and the development of talent. In R. Sternberg & J. Davidson (Eds.), *Conceptions of giftedness.* New York: Cambridge University Press.

Dweck, C.S., & Elliott, E.S. (1983). Achievement motivation. In P.H. Mussen (Ed.), *Handbook of child psychology* (pp. 643–691). New York: Wiley.

Edwards, B. (1979). *Drawing on the right side of the brain: a course in enhancing creativity and artistic confidence.* Los Angeles: J.P. Tarcher; Boston: Houghton-Mifflin.

Feldman, D.H. (1980). *Beyond universals in cognitive development.* Norwood: Ablex.

Feldman, D.H. (1986). *Nature's gambit.* New York: Basic Books.

Fodor, J. (1983). *The modularity of mind.* Cambridge: MIT Press.

Gardner, H. (1983). *Frames of mind: The theory of multiple intelligences.* New York: Basic Books.

Gardner, H. (1990a). The difficulties of school: Probable causes, possible cures. *Daedalus, 119,* 85–113.

Gardner, H. (1990b). Assessment in context: The alternative to standardized testing. In B. Gifford (Ed.), *Report of the Commission on Testing and Public Policy.* Boston: Kluwer.

Goldman, J., Krechevsky, M., Meyaard, J., & Gardner, H. (1988). A developmental study of children's practical intelligence for school. Harvard Project Zero Technical Report.

Hyde, A., & Bizar, M. (1989). *Thinking in context: Teaching cognitive processes across the elementary school curriculum.* New York: Longman.

Nisbet, J. (1989). Background paper presented at the International Conference of the Centre for Educational Research and Innovation, 'The curriculum redefined: Learning to think – Thinking to learn', Paris, France.

Palincsar, A.S., & Brown, A.L. (1984). Reciprocal teaching of comprehension-fostering and monitoring activities. *Cognition and Instruction, 1,* 117–175.

Perkins, D.N., & Salomon, G. (1989). Are cognitive skills context-bound? *Educational Researcher, 18,* 16–25.

Resnick, L. (1987). Learning in school and out. *Educational Researcher, 16,* 13–20.

Rogoff, B., & Lave, J. (Eds.) (1984). *Everyday cognition: Its development in social context.* Cambridge: Harvard University Press.

Schoenfeld, A.H. (1988). Problem solving in context(s). In R.I. Charles & E.A. Silver (Eds.), *The teaching and assessing of mathematical problem solving.* Reston: National Council of Teachers of Mathematics.

Scribner, S., & Cole, M. (1973). Cognitive consequences of formal and informal education. *Science, 182,* 553–559.

Sternberg, R.J. (1985). *Beyond IQ: A triarchic theory of human intelligence.* New York: Cambridge University Press.

Sternberg, R.J. (1988). *The triarchic mind.* New York: Viking.

Strauss, C. (1988). Culture, discourse, and cognition: Forms of beliefs in some Rhode Island working men's talk about success. Unpublished doctoral dissertation, Harvard University.

Strauss, S. (Ed.) (1982). *U-Shaped behavioral growth.* New York: Academic Press.

Wagner, D.A., & Stevenson, H.W. (Eds.) (1982). *Cultural perspectives on child development.* San Francisco: Freeman.

Wiggins, G. (1989). A true test: Toward more authentic and equitable assessment. *Phi Delta Kappa, 70,* 703–713.

Kuhn D (ed): Developmental Perspectives on Teaching and Learning Thinking Skills.
Contrib Hum Dev. Basel, Karger, 1990, vol 21, pp 95–107

Social Relations and Children's Thinking Skills

William Damon

My message in this chapter is simply stated. Children learn thinking skills through activities that require thinking, and such activities typically arise from the key social relations in a child's life. When so stated, this message may sound self-evident. It is also a message that is thoroughly shopworn, embedded in old pedagogical theories like Dewey's and Piaget's as well as in more current approaches like 'activity theory' and 'situated' cognition [Brown et al., 1989]. Yet despite both its apparentness and its longevity, it is not a message that has had much lasting influence on traditional schooling [Cremin, 1964; Graham, 1981].

Historians of education may have answers to why schools have resisted a focus on children's thinking skills, or to why schools have not made better use of children's key social relations in the educational enterprise. Whatever the traditional forces that have prevented such efforts, they are very much in effect today – as witness the popular appeal of the Hirsch 'cultural literacy' lists of what 'every schoolchild should know' [Hirsch, 1987]. It seems that advocates of thinking never have been able to make their cases either to the general public or to the educational establishment that it supports.

But this chapter is not about educational history or politics. It is an attempt to show how an action-oriented, social-relational framework can help us understand and foster children's thinking skills. Such a framework, I believe, derives directly from developmental theory and research, though it departs in important ways from the more typical cognitivist writings on thinking. It is also a framework that addresses the most pressing problem of schooling today, children's motivation to learn. I do not know whether a social-relational approach will be more likely than any other focus on thinking to gain acceptance into the mainstream of public schooling. My hope is that it will, because, when fully articulated, a social-relational approach could offer us a realistic strategy for orienting schoolchildren towards thinking and learning. In this chapter I take some beginning steps towards such an articulation.

Interactional Diversity and Developmental Outcome

The core assumption of a social-relational approach is that children bring away from their social interactions a number of cognitive products. The most noticeable of these products is the knowledge which children may acquire through discourse of one kind or another. While communicating with others, children learn facts about the world, they learn to speak, they learn values, they learn how to accomplish various tasks, and so on. But in addition to knowledge, children also learn procedures of thinking from social discourse. For example, through the social process of asking and answering questions, they learn to question themselves. This opens the door to fundamental intellectual functions of verification. Similarly, children learn basic mental processes like justification, invention, and logic itself from their participation in social communication. This social-relational assumption has appeared in the writings of developmentalists for generations [Baldwin, 1902; Werner and Kaplan, 1963; Piaget, 1966], but it has been most clearly explicated in Vygotskian theory [Wertsch, 1987].

Corollary to this social-relational assumption, but rarely explored, is the notion that the nature of a child's social interactions is linked to the nature of the cognitive products arising from those interactions. In other words, not only do social relations create the context for cognitive growth, but they also determine, by their nature, the nature of the cognitive growth that ensues. This becomes a strong claim when we begin to make qualitative distinctions between key types of social interaction. In a child's life, as in everyone's, there are many qualitatively distinct patterns of social interaction. The claim here is that different patterns may be associated with different types of cognitive acquisition.

Where do these distinct patterns themselves come from? To some extent, the nature of a social interaction derives from its specific social-relational context. A friendship, for example, spawns different sorts of interactions than a bitter rivalry. All important social relationships have a character of their own, deriving from their adaptive functions, as well as from their own histories. Specific interactions within relationships can never be independent of this overarching character [Hinde, 1979]. As a consequence, a relationship will always shape the distinct quality of the interactions that compose it.

In the psychological literature, much has been made of the distinction between adult/child and child/child relations [Youniss, 1980; Hartup, 1979]. Not only are these two archtypical childhood relations seen to be qualitatively distinct, but, as a direct consequence of their distinctness, they are seen to leave different sorts of developmental legacies. If this indeed is the case, it is an example of how social relations with particular functions give rise to social interactions of a particular nature. In turn, each type of social interaction engenders a particular type of cognitive product. I return to this example in more detail below.

Not every qualitative mark of a social interaction, however, is determined by its broad social-relational context. Whether the child is communicating with an adult or with a peer does not tell us everything we need to know about the nature of the communication. Sometimes an adult will speak to a child like a friend. Other times a peer will act like a boss. Moreover, there are many disparate ways of acting like a friend and acting like a boss. Each of these ways may have its own developmental implications for those who act them out. As a rule, the qualities of a social exchange that foster learning are as much interaction-specific as they are relationship-determined. Both factors need to be considered for a full understanding of the social contributors to children's thinking.

Varieties of Adult-Child Learning Interactions

Most adult-child interactions reflect a fundamental asymmetry. It is the adult, not the child, who directs the course of the interaction. This asymmetry follows naturally from the adult's greater competence, knowledge, and power, all of which are usually recognized by both adult and child. In most adult-child relations, adult direction is the dominant interactional quality, at least until the time the child makes credible claims to equal status. Even then, the transition to other interactional patterns can be bumpy and uncertain, as witness the agitation of the teenage years.

The asymmetry and adult-directedness of adult-child interactions create a particular kind of context for learning. Like all contexts for learning, it is one that has potential advantages and disadvantages for the child. Its primary advantage is that it provides the best available means of transmitting the culture's accumulated store of knowledge to the developing child. In an adult-child instructional communication, the adult represents what is known. If the communication is effective, the child comes away with some part of this established knowledge. A working understanding of the cultural heritage is thereby passed on from one generation to the next. Accompanying this transmitted understanding, according to some theorists, is an ancillary respect for the existing order of things [Piaget, 1965; Youniss, 1980]. This respect, however, may lead to certain cognitive imbalances, such as an uncritical acceptance of the adult word and an overreliance on imitation as a means of learning new skills. The very strengths of an interactional pattern thus define its developmental limitations.

Although most adult-child interactions have certain things in common – their asymmetries of status, for example – there are also many variations within and among them. Adults have many distinct ways of assuming leading roles in their dealing with children. These may have critical implications for the kinds of learning that takes place between child and adult. Consider a contrast between two such ways. The first is direct lecturing, as when an adult simply tells a child something (Ottawa is the capital of Canada; the area of a rectangle is the height times the width; stealing is against the law because people have a right to keep their own property). The second is reciprocal communication, established through leading questions, collaborative activities, and inductive reasoning. Here the adult implements an instructional plan by encouraging the child to actively help solve the problem. This second strategy is as old as planned pedagogy itself. It has been most commonly known as the Socratic method. Educational research has introduced many new variants to this second form of adult-child interaction – discovery learning, reciprocal teaching, guided participation, and so on [Hawkins, 1974; Palincsar and Brown, 1985; Rogoff, 1986], and each of these variants had its own special properties. In comparing direct lecturing and reciprocal communication, I shall not attempt to preserve the many important distinctions among such variants – even though potentially (by the same logic on which this chapter is founded), any of these distinctions could make a powerful difference for the child's learning.

By definition, direct lecturing and reciprocal communication create very different interaction patterns between adult and child. The former relies on the adult's skills as message-maker as well as on the child's somewhat passive attentiveness. The latter relies on the ability of the adult to create a joint activity and guide it toward an instructional goal, and on the child's ability to participate in the activity and eventually to share the goal.

In her writings on 'guided participation', Rogoff [1986] suggests five qualities that, to a greater or lesser extent, distinguish a reciprocal communication mode of instruction from a direct lecturing one. Guided participation

(1) Provides a bridge between familiar skills or information and those needed to solve a new problem; (2) provides a structure for problem solving; (3) involves the transfer of responsibility for management of problem solving; (4) involves active participation by the child as well as the adult; (5) may be tacit as well as explicit in the everyday arrangements and interactions between adults and children [Rogoff, 1986, p. 86].

Although each of these interactional qualities is found more often in reciprocal communication than in direct lecturing, qualities 3 and 4 are the ones that most clearly distinguish the reciprocal mode.

What is the significance of such distinctions for children's learning? Despite centuries of educational theorizing around such issues, there has yet to be a conclusive empirical test comparing the learning effects of direct lecturing to those of reciprocal communication. Nevertheless, the theorizing gives us some grounds to speculate. Based on the interactional nature of the two patterns, it is reasonable to suspect that, while certain information may be transmitted more efficiently through direct lecturing, many cognitive and metacognitive skills are more readily attained through reciprocal communication. This is so because, unlike direct lecturing, reciprocal communication engages children in the social equivalents of critical thinking processes. It is precisely this kind of engagement that leads the child's toward the acquisition of these thinking processes.

A number of developmental models account for how this transformation from the social to the mental occurs. Certainly the most finely elaborated is Soviet-style activity theory [Wertsch, 1981; Vygotsky, 1978], a perspective based on the notion that children 'internalize' the dialogical features of their social interactions. There are, of course, competing process models, ranging from the neo-Piagetian to the social-psychological. For current purposes, the commonalities among these models are more germane than the contrasts. The key commonality is the core assumption: In the course of development, children's thinking tends to replicate the procedural logic of the social communications in which they participate. In fact, this tendency describes not only the direction of intellectual development but one of its primary determinants.

Specifically, the 'procedural logic' generated by a child's participation in social communication includes planning, verification, justification, explanation, evaluation, and criticism. These functions originate in social relationships and become essential components of critical thinking. Because they are both social and cognitive functions, they link the interpersonal plane with the individual. They are the most enduring part of what developing children 'bring away' with them from their social engagements. Hartup [1985] has called them the 'executive regulators', and consistent with my argument here, he has predicted that these are precisely the functions that constitute the cognitive 'derivatives' of children's social relations:

> ... the cognitive functions most closely linked to social relationships are the 'executive regulators' – the planning, monitoring, and outcome-checking skills involved in problem-solving ... (including) (a) predicting one's capacity limitations; (b) being aware of the repertoire that one has available for problem-solving; (c) identifying the problem; (d) planning with respect to strategy; (e) monitoring the routines one uses; (f) evaluating outcomes; and (g) using them to make adjustments in one's activities [Hartup, 1985, p. 76].

It is clear why reciprocal communications between adults and children provide an optimal relational format for inducing these cognitive regulators. As Rogoff's [1986] ethnographic observations show, during such activity adults commonly help children identify problems, predict their limitations, build upon the problem-solving skills they already have, create plans and subplans, monitor their progress, and evaluate the result. It is a direct (though not by any means immediate) developmental step from engaging in these adult-initiated activities during social discourse to acquiring the capacity to perform these same activities during individual mentation.

In Rogoff's observations, it is the mother-child dyad that provides the prototype. Hartup too suggests that the mother-child relation provides an interaction pattern especially well-suited for generating executive cognitive functions. Hartup's reasons are illuminating: Mothers know their children well and are therefore good at building communicational bridges that take account of the child's strengths and weaknesses. The question remains, though, as to whether mothers typically have instructional (rather than immediate, task-oriented) goals in mind when they interact with their children. Recent studies have shown that not much learning takes place unless the mother not only shares task responsibility with the child but also guides the child towards a cognitive achievement of some sort – that is, an achievement beyond the actual task that mother and child are working on together [Gauvain and Rogoff, 1989; Gauvain, 1989]. In other words, the adult must guide the interaction toward some implicit or explicit instructional agenda. On this score, teachers may be better prepared than mothers to provide the best sustained guidance.

Whether it is parent, teacher, or some other adult directing the interaction, it is the quality of the interaction itself that determines what the child learns. No doubt there are many ways to learn new facts and information. But the central procedures of thinking, including most prominently the 'executive functions' identified above, follow most readily from certain key qualities of the interaction. Among these is the quality of adult directedness. A peer cannot be expected to engage a fellow peer in the systematic guidance needed for the acquisition of planning and other executive skills. But adult directedness, while necessary, is not sufficient in itself. Also required is an opportunity for the child to engage in reciprocal communication with the guiding adult – and, for maximum effect, a clear instructional agenda on the part of the adult.

These interactional qualities facilitate learning in both the intellectual and social spheres. Baumrind's [1989] findings on the effects of authoritative child rearing, for example, show that adult-guided interactions with frequent reciprocal communications are far more likely to generate social responsibility on the part of the child than are either non-guided (permissive) or non-reciprocal (authoritarian) interactions. The developmental processes in the social sphere are the same as those in the intellectual sphere. In order to acquire internal regulators of thought and action, the child needs to participate actively in relations that introduce the child to external forms of such regulators. Over time and development, the regulators become part of the child's own system of executive controls. Such controls establish an autonomous sense of social responsibility in one's personal life just as they establish critical thinking in one's intellectual life [Damon, 1988].

Varieties of Peer Interaction and Their Diverse Contributions to Children's Learning

Over the past 10 years, the research communities in education and developmental psychology have awakened to the possibility that peer relations are not always a negative influence on children's academic learning. Literally hundreds of studies have explored experimental uses of peer interaction in education. Some of the new peer-based techniques have found their way into the classroom, and increasingly teachers are expected to know something about cooperative learning as part of their pedagogical repertoire. (See, for example, the new NASDAC standards for teacher certification.)

It is interesting, therefore, to note how peer learning is actually implemented in a typical classroom. The following observation comes from Kidder's 1989 book, *Among schoolchildren.* The teacher, Chris Zajac, is portrayed throughout the book as a dedicated and reasonably enlightened teacher.

> Then came 15 minutes of study, during which teams of two children quizzed each other. Chris paired up good spellers with poor ones. She also made spelling an exercise in socialization, by putting together children who did not seem to like each other. She hoped that some would learn to get along with children that they didn't think they liked. At least they'd be more apt to do some work than if she paired them up with friends [Kidder, 1989, p. 114].

In arranging a peer learning experience for her pupils, Ms. Zajac has made several significant choices. These choices will determine the quality of pupils' interaction and, as I have argued throughout this chapter, the quality of their interaction will determine the kinds of learning that take place during their engagement.

Three of Ms. Zajac's choices strike me as particularly consequential: (1) she focuses on the peer engagements around the subject matter of spelling; (2) she pairs more competent children with less competent ones; and (3) she constructs the dyads of children who are not friends. All of these choices seem to be intentional. My guess is that Ms. Zajac chooses spelling because it is a peripheral subject and therefore one that can be given less of her direct attention; during part of the peer spelling exercise she retreats to the teacher's lounge for a break. Ms. Zajac puts good spellers together with poor ones so that the former can teach the latter something. And she refrains from putting friends together on the assumption that children cannot be trusted to engage in serious learning tasks with children that they like a lot.

Whatever their intuitive merits, these choices are not well informed by educational research. Starting with the last issue, there is plenty of evidence that close friendships are conducive, rather than inimical, to serious peer learning. In fact, the closer the friendship, the better the joint performance, the richer the interaction, and the greater the learning benefit [Berndt, 1989]. As for subject matter, spelling skills have been one area in which peer formats have been used with some success and, like Ms. Zajac, researchers generally have paired more with less competent children when teaching spelling through peer interaction [Allen, 1976]. But educational research has uncovered more central applications of peer-based instruction. Most of these applications rely on children working together as partners with equal rather than unequal competence. Many researchers believe that equality in a peer relation is itself an interactional characteristic that facilitates communication and therefore learning [Berndt and Ladd, 1989]. Others believe that progress is best fostered through equal but distinct role relations that divide tasks across a variety of clearly defined responsibilities [Cohen, 1986]. The unequal 'peer tutoring' mode is just one of several available peer arrangements that educators may use in their classrooms, but its characteristic of inequality severely limits the use to which it may be put.

Like adult-child relations, peer relations vary widely in their interactional characteristics. As in adult-child relations, these variations make a difference for children's learning. In previous writings [Damon, 1989; Damon and Phelps, 1989], I have distinguished three types of peer learning arrangement – peer tutoring, cooperative learning, and peer collaboration. In peer tutoring, one child instructs another on material in which the former is more competent than the latter. Sometimes the tutor is older than the tutee; it is common to pair sixth graders with first graders, for example. But at other times (as in Ms. Zajac's class) tutor and tutee come from the same grade. In cooperative learning, a team of children work together on a single task. Usually the teacher divides the task into separate subcomponents, the students are assigned different problem-solving roles, they work independently on their own assignments, and they report back to the team. The children are assumed to have equal competence despite their separate problem-solving roles. In peer collaboration, a pair of children work together on challenging tasks that neither child would be able to solve prior to their learning engagement. In contrast to peer tutoring, the children begin at roughly the same level of competence. In contrast to cooperative learning, the children at all times work jointly on the same aspects of the problem and communicate constantly with one another. As in my discussion of adult-child interaction patterns, these are ideal-type descriptions that are not always represented purely in practice. There are important variations within each of the three approaches, as well as many shades of grey between them. Some techniques blend aspects of more than one approach, particularly with respect to cooperative learning and peer collaboration.

The three types of interaction can in principle be distinguished from one another by comparing the extent to which they embody two central dimensions of peer discourse, equality and mutuality of engagement. Mutuality in a relationship implies an extensive, intimate, and 'connected' engagement – 'the degree to which children are involved in a conversation and "in tune" with one another' [Berndt, 1989]. Although equality and mutuality are basic dimensions for all peer relations, the three types of peer learning reflect these dimensions quite differently. Peer tutoring is relatively low on equality and high on mutuality; cooperative learning is high on equality and varied on mutuality (depending on the specific technique used); and peer collaboration is high on both.

There are sound theoretical reasons, and a growing body of empirical evidence, in support of the idea that these differences determine the kinds of learning that take place within the three peer arrangements. Developmental theory would predict that the particular combination of equality and mutuality represented in each arrangement should foster a particular form of intellectual achievement. Peer tutoring, with its low equality and high mutuality, should lead to the mastering of ideas that can be readily transmitted through direct lecturing and practice. The peer tutor instructs and drills the tutee in 'packaged' sets of knowledge and skills. Accuracy and adeptness – in spelling, computation, word recognition, and so on – may be facilitated, but basic concepts and important new insights are not likely to be acquired in this way. In contrast, the pattern of high equality and high mutuality in peer collaboration offers a supportive 'discovery learning' context in which genuinely new insights and skills may be generated. One would not expect, however, that this would be the best way to pass on comprehensive or even accurate representations of 'what is known'. This contrast between the learning effects of tutoring and collaborative engagements conforms to theoretical distinctions often proposed by developmentalists [Piaget, 1932; Youniss, 1980; Doise and Mugny, 1984;

Kroger and Tomasello, 1986]. These distinctions apply as well to the variations among existing cooperative learning approaches; some have features similar to peer collaborations, whereas others look more like tutoring or some mix of the two [Damon and Phelps, 1989].

Empirically, there is evidence that collaborative forms of cooperative learning arrangements are more likely than peer tutoring arrangements to foster basic concepts and higher-order reasoning skills [Slavin, 1980; Sharan, 1984]. Conversely, peer tutoring has been shown to be a good inducer of competence in multiplication tables, spelling, interacting with a computer, reciting historical facts, 'word attack' skills, and other practice-based intellectual abilities. In our own research, we have not directly compared peer collaboration and peer tutoring, but we have explored the learning constraints of collaborative arrangements [Damon and Phelps, 1989; Phelps and Damon, in press]. We have found that, in the math and science area, peer collaboration can foster the acquisition of dramatic new insights about basic concepts such as proportionality and spatial relations – concepts that are notoriously difficult to teach to children directly. In contrast, we did not find significant learning effects of peer collaboration on tasks requiring replication of models or formulaic arithmetic calculations. Such tasks, of course, rely on readily transmittable information rather than on deep conceptual shifts in one's own thinking.

Conclusions

The message from the peer studies is the same as that from the adult-child studies: Interactional patterns vary within and among relationships, and these variations are linked to predictable differences in the learning outcomes of the relationships. We are only beginning to unearth all the interactional variations that have implications for learning and to understand what these implications are. But it is already clear that a comprehensive approach to children's learning must be socially pluralistic – that is, it must employ the full diversity of learning contexts that play a role in intellectual development.

It is not enough simply to compare one relational format against another. Each of the instructional patterns that we have considered – direct lecturing and reciprocal communication between adult and child, and the three distinct forms of peer education – has its strengths and limitations. Some are more appropriate for conveying information, others for encouraging practice and mastery, still others for stimulating conceptual revision and autonomous thought. Differences may also exist in the extent to which each can contribute to learning within a particular discipline. Certainly there are important motivational advantages and disadvantages of each as well. The agenda for both research and educational practice is to identify the special instructional potential of all the social relations and interactional patterns in children's lives. We may then determine which of them meet our goals for schooling; and children's thinking skills should be high on our lists of goals. If, as a consequence, schools come to use a diversity of social relations to enrich children's thinking, we shall find that we have stretched our notions of schooling more than a bit. We also may have stretched the learning potential of children in the process.

References

Allen, V.L. (1976). *Children as teachers: Theory and research on tutoring.* New York: Academic Press.

Baldwin, J.M. (1902). *Social and ethical interpretations in mental development.* New York: Macmillan.

Baumrind, D. (1989). Rearing competent children. In W. Damon (Ed.), *Child development today and tomorrow.* San Francisco: Jossey-Bass.

Berndt, T., & Ladd, G. (Eds.) (1989). *Peer relationships in child development.* New York: Wiley.

Berndt, T. (1989). Contributions of peer relations to children's development. In T. Berndt & G. Ladd (Eds.), *Peer relationships in child development.* New York: Wiley.

Brown, J.S., Collins, A., & Duguid, P. (1989). Situated cognition and the culture of learning. *Educational researcher, 18,* 32–42.

Cohen, E.G. (1986). *Designing groupwork: Strategies for the heterogenous classroom.* New York: Teachers Colllege Press.

Cremin, L.A. (1964). *The transformation of the school: Progressivism in American education.* New York: Knopf.

Damon, W. (1984). Peer-based education: The untapped potential. *Journal of Applied Developmental Psychology, 5,* 331–343.

Damon, W., & Phelps, E. (1989). Critical distinctions among three forms of peer learning. *International Journal of Educational Research, 13,* 9–19.

Doise, W., & Mugny, G. (1984). *The social development of the intellect.* New York: Pergamon.

Gauvain, M. (1989). Influence of knowledge of a posttest and child age on adult-child planning. Paper presented at the biannual meeting of the Society for Research in Child Development, Kansas City.

Gauvain, M., & Rogoff, B. (1989). Collaborative problem solving and children's planning skills. *Developmental Psychology, 25,* 139–151.

Graham, P.A. (1981). American education and the schools. *Daedalus, 154,* 56–89.

Hartup, W.W. (1979). The social worlds of childhood. *American Psychologist, 34,* 944–950.

Hartup, W.W. (1985). Relationships and their significance in cognitive development. In R.A. Hinde, A. Perret-Clermont, & J. Stevenson-Hinde (Eds.), *Social relationships and cognitive development.* Oxford: Clarendon Press.

Hawkins, D. (1974). *The informed vision.* Cambridge: Harvard University Press.

Hinde, R.A. (1979). *Towards understanding relationships.* London: Academic Press.

Hirsch, E.D., Jr. (1987). *Cultural literacy: What every American needs to know.* New York: Vintage.

Kidder, T. (1989). *Among schoolchildren.* Boston: Houghton Mifflin.

Kruger, A.C., & Tomasello, M. (1986). Transactive discussions with peers and adults. *Developmental Psychology, 22,* 681–685.

Palincsar, A., & Brown, A. (1985). Reciprocal teaching of comprehension-fostering and comprehension-monitoring activities. *Cognition and Instruction, 1,* 117–175.

Phelps, E., & Damon, W. (in press). Promoting change in children's math and science conceptions through peer collaboration. *Journal of Educational Psychology.*

Piaget, J. (1965). *The moral judgment of the child.* New York: Free Press.

Piaget, J. (1966). *Etudes sociologiques.* Geneva: Droz.

Rogoff, B. (1986). Adult assistance of children's learning. In T.E. Raphael (Ed.), *The contexts of school-based literacy.* New York: Random House.

Sharon, S. (1984). *Cooperative learning.* Hillsdale: Erlbaum.

Slavin, R. (1980). A review of peer tutoring and cooperative learning projects in twenty-eight schools. *Review of Educational Research, 11,* 315–342.

Vygotsky, L.S. (1978). *Mind in society: The development of higher psychological processes.* Cambridge MA: Harvard University Press.

Wertsch, J. (1981). *The concept of activity in Soviet Psychology.* Armonk: Sharpe.

Werner, H., & Kaplan, B. (1963). *Symbol formation.* New York: Wiley.

Wertsch, J. (1985). *Vygotsky and the social formation of mind.* Cambridge MA: Harvard University Press.

Youniss, J. (1980). *Parents and peers in social development: a Sullivan-Piaget perspective.* Chicago: University of Chicago Press.

Kuhn D (ed): Developmental Perspectives on Teaching and Learning Thinking Skills.
Contrib Hum Dev. Basel, Karger, 1990, vol 21, pp 108–126

Communities of Learning and Thinking, or A Context by Any Other Name

Ann L. Brown, Joseph C. Campione

Why Johnny can't read was one of the central questions raised about American education in the 1970s. Why Johnny can't think replaced it in the 1980s. In the last decade, interest in how one might teach students to think more critically has increased for both pragmatic and theoretical reasons [Glaser, 1984; Resnick, 1987; Segal, Chipman, and Glaser, 1985]. American schools in the latter part of the 20th century face dramatic change in the population they must serve, at the same time that the demands of the workplace require complex forms of literacy – those that go beyond simple rote acts of reading and calculating. Increasingly, educated graduates need to be able to critically evaluate what they read, express themselves clearly in verbal and written forms, understand scientific and mathematical thinking, and be comfortable with various forms of technology that can serve as tools for thinking. Schools are required to foster high literacy [Resnick and Resnick, 1977] aimed at developing students' reasoning [Miller, 1988], rather than the low literacies of minimum competence that now serve as exit criteria. And, in addition to the basic competencies of literacy, numeracy and computer familiarity, we would also like students to acquire integrated and usable knowledge, rather than sets of compartmentalized facts rarely applied to novel situations. In short, we would like our graduates to be independent, self-motivated critical thinkers able to take responsibility for life-long learning. Easier said than done!

Although the need to foster these so called higher-order thinking skills is clearly recognized, there is considerable debate about how one might achieve this end [Resnick, 1987]. Principally, the controversy has focused on the domain generality or specificity of thinking skills, with the corollary problem of whether to teach thinking skills in the context of academic subject matter or as a separate domain. Opinions range from those who specifically design instructional material that is independent of traditional academic domains [Feuerstein, 1980] to those who argue that thinking skills are an integral part of a domain of inquiry and cannot be taught outside of the context of that domain. For example, Schoenfeld [1985] argues that one cannot follow Polya's [1945] advice on how to improve one's mathematical problem-solving skills unless one is already a quite knowledgeable mathematician. It is also possible to hold to the middle ground and argue that skills of wide applicability can be acquired within recognizable academic pursuits, such as reading, and it is this approach that we have followed.

A second area of controversy has been provoked by the use of the term *higher-order* thinking skills to describe reasoning. Higher-order thinking skills are often contrasted to basic skills, leading to the perception that such entities are not for all. Younger and more disadvantaged students are held accountable for basic skills, whereas higher-order thinking skills are seen as part of upper school curricula or, worse still, optional extras. We argue that this is absurd; thinking and reasoning should be part of the curriculum from the earliest years, and indeed fostering effective reasoning should be the main responsibility of schools. Ideally, students should develop a belief system based on rationality and sensitivity to evidence; they should acquire a general attitude to learning that is based on reasoning in all areas of the curriculum and from the earliest age. It is for this reason that our work has primarily addressed academically at-risk elementary school children.

For several years, we have been studying the reading comprehension activities of academically marginal children. The decision to target reading as a domain in which to foster critical thinking in children followed from two pragmatic considerations. First, reading is the primary achievement required in elementary school. It is failure in reading in the earliest grades that singles out children for labelling and remedial intervention and all that entails. If one could 'inoculate' students against failure in the early grades by enhancing reading, the result might be that their future academic trajectories would prove more promising. Second, disadvantaged students, perhaps because of their greater need of basic skills instruction, are more likely to be subjected to practice in disaggregated skills that lack meaning and coherence. The problem is exacerbated by the tradition of 'pulling out' children for supplementary instruction that consists overwhelmingly of skills practice; comprehension practice if provided at all, is left up to the regular classroom teacher. Given that students cannot perfect what they do not practice, our aim was to provide that practice with respect to comprehension.

In this chapter, we describe the history of our research program on reading to learn in a variety of contexts. We began by considering the traditional reading group as the context of thinking instruction, but became increasingly dissatisfied with the ecological validity of the reading group as a forum for learning, at least in the later grades. Our more recent work concentrates on classrooms as communities of learning where critical thinking is practiced in the service of learning coherent content.

Higher-Order Thinking Skills in Reading

Texts are a major source of information available to a literate society. In order to enter that society fully, students must know how to learn from reading. Much of what is called reading in the later grades is indistinguishable from critical thinking and studying. Students are not only required to decode, they are also required to understand the meaning, critically evaluate the message, remember the content, and apply the new-found knowledge flexibly and creatively. The premium placed on understanding and using information gleaned from texts increases through the high school and college years when texts, to a large extent, take the place of teachers as the primary source of knowledge. Students who have not honed the necessary critical reading skills suffer a considerable and cumulative disadvantage.

More than ever before, schools must equip people to deal with facts that they never encountered in school. In a scientific and technological society based on an increasingly complex and rapidly changing information base, a productive member of society must be able to acquire new facts, evaluate them critically, and adapt to their implications. Reliance on remembered facts and fallacies from outmoded past schooling will not suffice. Schools, therefore, need to develop *intelligent novices* [Brown et al., 1983]. Intelligent novices are those who, although they may not possess the background knowledge needed in a new field, know how to go about gaining that knowledge. Intelligent novices have learned how to learn from texts, rather than merely to memorize facts.

Considerable evidence exists that a sizable minority of school leavers, when they encounter college, the armed forces, or the workplace, lack the skills of the intelligent novice. Questioned about their preferred study strategies, high school students vary in their sophistication. For example, one student claimed that when called upon to study, ' ... I stare real hard at the page, blink my eyes and then open them – and cross my fingers that it will be right here' (pointing at his head). A somewhat better informed peer replied, 'It's easy; if she (the teacher) says study, I read it twice. If she says read, it's just once through'. A third answered, 'I just read the first line in each paragraph – it's usually all there'. These are not expert readers.

In contrast, intelligent novices possess a wide repertoire of strategies for gaining new knowledge from texts. Critical reading demands a divided mental focus whereby readers both concentrate on acquiring knowledge and simultaneously monitor their level of understanding. These 'metacognitive skills' of reading include: (a) clarifying the purposes of reading, i.e., understanding the task demands, both explicit and implicit; (b) spontaneously making use of relevant background knowledge; (c) allocating attention so that concentration can be focused on the major content at the expense of trivia; (d) critically evaluating content for internal consistency and compatibility with prior knowledge and common sense; (e) monitoring ongoing activities to see if comprehension is occurring, by engaging in such activities as periodic self-review; (f) drawing and testing inferences of many kinds, including interpretations, predictions, and conclusions; and (g) criticizing, refining, and extending the newly acquired knowledge by imagining other uses of the information or counterexamples to the arguments. In short, reading is thinking, and thinking demands effort and skill [Brown, 1980]. Our research question then became how to lead students who don't read critically in that direction.

Fostering Reading Comprehension via Reciprocal Teaching

We have been involved in a program for promoting reading comprehension, termed reciprocal teaching [Brown and Palincsar, 1989], for almost a decade. Briefly, reciprocal teaching is a procedure that features guided practice in applying simple concrete strategies to the task of text comprehension. An adult teacher and a group of students take turns 'being the teacher', i.e., leading a discussion about material that they have either read silently or listened to the adult teacher reading. The learning leader (adult or child) begins the discussion by asking a question and ends by summarizing the gist of what has been learned. Questioning provides the impetus to get the discussion going. Summarizing at the end of a period of discussion helps students establish where they are in preparation for tackling a new segment of text. Attempts to clarify any comprehension problems that might arise occur opportunistically when someone misunderstands, or does not know the meaning of a concept, word, or phrase, etc. And, finally, the leader asks for predictions about future content if this is appropriate.

We lack space to go into the theoretical rationale for reciprocal teaching in detail, but we will make several points. First, the strategies (questioning, clarifying, summarizing, and predicting) were not randomly chosen. They are excellent cognitive monitoring devices; if one cannot summarize what one has read, it is an excellent indication that understanding is not proceeding smoothly and remedial action is required. The strategies also provide the repeatable structure necessary to get a discussion going.

Second, the cooperative feature of the learning groups is an essential feature. The group is jointly responsible for understanding and evaluating the text. All members of the group, in turn, serve as learning leaders, the ones responsible for guiding the dialogue, and as learning listeners, those whose job is to encourage the discussion leader to explain the content and help resolve misunderstandings. The goal is joint construction of meaning. The reciprocal nature of the procedure forces student engagement. Teacher modeling provides examples of expert performance. Everyone is seeking consensus concerning meaning, relevance, and importance. The setting is ideal for novices to practice their emergent comprehension skills. All of the responsibility for comprehending does not rest with one person, and even if a learning leader falters, the other members of the group, including the adult teacher, are there to keep the discussion going. Because the group's efforts are externalized in the form of a discussion, novices can learn from the contributions of those more expert than they. It is in this sense that reciprocal teaching sessions create a zone of proximal development [Vygotsky, 1978] for their participants; all may share in the co-construction of meaning to the extent that they are able. Collaboratively, the group, with its variety of goals, expertise, and engagement gets the job done; the text gets understood. What changes over time is who has the major responsibility for the learning activities.

Third, the adult teacher plays many roles. She (1) models expert behavior; (2) monitors the group's understanding; (3) engages in on-line diagnosis of emerging competence; (4) pushes for deeper understanding; (5) scaffolds the weaker students' emerging competence; and (6) fades into the background whenever the students are able to take charge of their own learning.

The reciprocal teaching program has been used successfully as a reading and listening comprehension intervention by average classroom teachers with academically at-risk elementary and middle-school children. For example, between 1981 and 1987, 287 junior high-school and 366 early elementary-school children took part in reading and listening comprehension experiments. The teachers worked with small groups. (The ideal group size is six, but teachers have handled much larger groups.) Students enter the study with scores of approximately 30% correct on independent tests of text comprehension. Successful students achieve independent scores of 75–80% correct on five successive tests. Using this criterion, approximately 80% of students at both ages are successful. Furthermore, students maintain their independent mastery for up to a year after instruction ceases; the listening practice transfers to reading; students generalize to other classroom activities, notably science and social studies; and they improve approximately two years on standardized tests of reading comprehension. The program is in widespread use nationally, but we have no means of evaluating the interventions that are outside our control. We do know that under experimental conditions, reciprocal teaching produces results far in excess of other feasible instructional strategies featuring the key activities [Brown and Palincsar, 1989].

Reciprocal Teaching of Coherent Content

In the majority of our work on reciprocal teaching of reading comprehension, we have followed the typical practice in American classrooms of 'reading group'. Each day children read a text that is rarely related to the previous texts. Passage follows passage with no coherent link between them. A passage about volcanos might follow one on dinosaurs, that follows a description of aquanauts, two poems and a fairy tale. Clearly, there is little opportunity for cumulative reference, little opportunity for learning. The students are very much *learning to read* rather than *reading to learn.* Such procedures positively encourage the child to acquire encapsulated 'inert' knowledge [Whitehead, 1916], rarely accessed again or used to facilitate new learning. In contrast, mature reading in academic contexts demands reading of coherent content that builds successively on prior reading. It enables students to accumulate successively richer representations of a domain, applying principles of learning via analogy, example, explanation, and plausible reasoning based on gradually accumulating knowledge. Traditional 'reading group' practices effectively preclude such learning.

Our first attempt to remedy this situation was to maintain the practice of 'reading group', reading a text a day, but to include passages that contained repeating themes so that cross-reference was at least possible [Brown et al., in press]. We asked 'at-risk' minority third graders (age 8) to read related passages about animal survival, concentrating on such mechanisms as camouflage, mimicry, protection from the elements, extinction, parasites, and natural pest control. These themes occurred repeatedly during the discussions and were also featured in the daily independent tests of comprehension.

Over 20 days of such discussions, there was a dramatic improvement in both comprehension processes and theme understanding. Reciprocal teaching groups improved daily independent comprehension scores from approximately 35% to 80% correct, compared to a variety of control groups that did not improve significantly. Even 12 months later, students maintained performance at 80% correct.

Each day the discussion and test passages contained some material that was analogous. For example, under the natural pest control theme, the children might discuss the manatees, large sea mammals, that moved inland, where they took to eating the water hyacinths that had previously clogged Florida's inland waterways. The manatees were welcomed by the residents because they provided a biological (rather than chemical) solution to an environmental problem. Immediately after discussing this example of a biological deterrent, the students answered questions about an analogous problem of how to rid a garden of mosquitos, their having read that (a) purple martins eat mosquitos, and (b) purple martins like to live in man-made bird houses. An observant child, Jeremy, responded:

> The house owner could build a home for purple martins at the bottom of the garden ... but I think *Raid* is best – but it's just like the manatees we talked about ... and the ladybugs eating the farmer's a- a- [*teacher:* aphids] right, aphids – we talked about that last week.

Regular practice greatly improved the ability to use analogous information to solve problems. Children began by noting few of the analogies, but, after several days, they were able to solve 90% of the analogous problems by cross reference to the discussion passages.

Children also increased their use of analogy as an explanatory mechanism in discussions. In one example [Brown et al., in press], from the natural pest control theme, a group of children readily understood why farmers use ladybugs to destroy harmful aphids. Twelve days later, they recognized the similarity of the ladybug theme to the usefulness of manatees that rid inland waterways of clogging weeds. And even one year later, students immediately recognized the similarity of lacewings and ladybugs as natural pest controllers.

Not only did the children remember how to conduct the reciprocal teaching dialogues, they also remembered the content. Asked to sort pictures of animals into the six themes, they could not comply before entering the study, relying on surface similarity as a basis of categorization. However, they scored 85% correct immediately after the study, and 82% correct one year later. Also, on both long- and short-term knowledge tests, children were able to classify novel exemplars of the themes and place them in appropriate habitats. Reciprocal teaching experience enables students both to learn a body of coherent, usable, knowledge and to develop a repertoire of strategies that will enable them to learn new content on their own.

Reciprocal Teaching in the Context of an Intentional Learning Environment

In our most recent extension of the comprehension fostering program, reciprocal teaching was only one feature of a radical restructuring of classroom activity. In fact, we took over total responsibility for the students' social studies program, three hours a week for the entire academic year. Students were 90 fifth and sixth graders (age 10–11) of a wide range of ability (approximately one-quarter were diagnosed as learning disabled). We deliberately set out to create an intentional learning environment [Bereiter and Scardamalia, 1989] where students had a great deal of control over their own learning [Brown, 1988].

What to Teach: A Biology Curriculum

To take seriously the notion that critical thinking should be directed toward an acknowledged learning goal, we set out to invite children to learn about a topic in which they would be prepared to invest considerable time and effort. Because we wanted students to develop skills of plausible reasoning about probable cause, we selected the basic biological concept of interdependence in nature as the basis of the curriculum (after interviewing 10-year-old children about their interests). Informally reviewing elementary school science texts, we were appalled at the random coverage of unrelated facts. Similar to reading texts but less excusable, they have the following flaws: (1) *Pseudonarrative style.* The 'stories' are often written in 'Disneyland' style with animals personified in such a way that it is difficult for children to distinguish fact from fiction. (2) *Assumed developmental sequences.* Skills are introduced from basic to more advanced according to a simplistic developmental sequence. For example, 6-year-olds might be required to categorize shapes and colors, 9-year-olds animals by habitats, and 13-year-olds vertebrates and invertebrates. No rationale is given for why shapes and colors prepare students for more advanced categorization, nor even a mention of the fact that this is why the young children are playing sorting games. Thus, the younger the children, the weaker the rationale for activities and the more fragmented the curriculum. (3) *Lack of cumulative reference.* There is a striking lack of cumulative reference (volcanoes following magnets, following a unit on friction, then the seasons, etc.). This lack of coherent theme or underlying principle all but precludes systematic knowledge-building based on analogy, example, principle, etc. It does not encourage sustained effort after meaning. (4) *Causal explanation.* More problematic still, presumably in order to conform to outmoded readability formulas, causal explanations are omitted, or are at best left enigmatic, positively encouraging concentration on facts (what happens?) rather than generative understanding (why or how does it happen?).

So we generated our own 'person-on-the-street' science curriculum for use in middle-school classrooms. After an introductory section on animal defense mechanisms that we know children enjoy, we introduced two large units based on the same recurrent theme – interdependence in nature. The first, *Adaptation,* consisted of the subtopics extinction, adaptation, endangered species, zoos and bioparks, and habitat management. The second unit, *Endangered Ecosystems,* consisted of the subtopics oceans (oil spills), garbage and hazardous waste, global warming, food chains and animal habitats, and food chains and human populations. The units were designed to invite students to come to think in terms of interrelated systems: (1) that animals and their environments form a closely knit system; (2) that perturbations in any part of the system will reverberate throughout; and (3) that one can predict such changes, even in the absence of explicit prior knowledge, by reasoning plausibly on the basis of incomplete knowledge [Collins et al., 1975].

How to Teach: The Collaborative Classroom

Students were involved in designing their own curriculum units. The basic idea was adapted from the Jigsaw Classroom [Aronson, 1978]. Students formed research groups covering the five subunits of each topic. We provided suitable materials (texts, articles, magazines, videos, and access to a library, plus adult guidance upon request). They prepared a booklet on their research subtopic (using a simplified version of Hypercard on Macintosh IIs), and then regrouped into learning groups made up of one member from each of the research groups. The expert from each research group was responsible for teaching other members of the learning group about his or her topic of expertise. Thus, the choice of a learning leader was based on expertise rather than random selection, as in the original reciprocal teaching work.

All children in the learning group are experts on one-fifth of the material, teach it to others, and prepare questions for the test that all will take on the complete unit. The students are involved in: (a) extensive reading in order to research their topic; (b) writing and revision to produce booklets from which to teach and to publish books covering the entire topic; and (c) computer use to publish, illustrate, and edit their booklets. In addition, a great deal of cognitive monitoring must take place in order for students to set priorities concerning what to include in their books, what to teach, what to test, how to explain, and so forth. They are reading, writing, and using computers in the service of learning.

In addition to improvement on standard tests of reading, writing, biological knowledge, and computer skill, dramatic qualitative improvement occurred in the thinking processes reflected in the discussions and in the writing samples. A detailed microgenetic study of selected individual students is underway. Here we give some general impressions of student progress.

Classroom Dialogues

One immediate outcome of the collaborative classroom is the development of a community of learners acquiring and sharing a common knowledge base. The nature of the reading/learning discussions and the writing samples all reflect higher levels of reasoning skills than were apparent in the original reciprocal teaching dialogues. Although children in the collaborative classroom were all trained in the comprehension-monitoring strategies (question, clarify, summarize, predict) of reciprocal teaching, these activities took on less and less importance as the argument and explanatory structure of the teaching sessions developed. Over time we saw an increasing incidence of comprehension-extending activities, such as deep analogies occurring in the teaching dialogues. A surface analogy is one in which students notice similarities across incidents but do not use them as explanatory devices; in contrast, deep analogies involve students not only noticing systematic relations but also using deep structural similarity to explain mechanisms. Similarly, causal explanations became more evident, again increasing in their explanatory precision and coherence over time. Explanations were more often supported by warrants and backings [Toulmin, 1958]. The nature of what constitutes evidence was discussed, including a consideration of negative evidence. A variety of plausible reasoning strategies [Collins et al., 1975] began to emerge. Argumentation formats developed, comparing different points of view and defensible interpretations. And finally, the nature and importance of prediction evolved, with students going beyond predictions of simple outcomes to considering possible worlds and engaging in thought experiments about what might happen in them. For example:

S_1: *(Question)* How long does it take man versus nature to make a species endangered?

S_2: If you're talking about endangered – well, say nature wanted to get rid of chameleons. The way nature would do it would be to change some of its colors so that chameleons couldn't fit in [couldn't disguise via camouflage], and the chameleons would die out. But people can just go out there and kill them in a day [destroy habitat]. But if nature caused it to die out, it would take many years because of all the changes.

In the first half of table 1, a group of children is discussing the new concepts of food chains and webs. They work long and hard and not all of them resolve the problem of the interdependence in the chain. The text doesn't help, as it depicts a top-down pyramid. In the second half of table 1, we see the same group three months later using the food chain notion quite well.

One of the main functions of the discussion is that students force each other to sort out their own misunderstandings. For example, in table 2, a

Table 1. Food chains and webs: excerpts from children's learning about food chains

---

S$_1$: *(Expert-question)* What is a food chain?

S$_2$: Um, it's like when bigger animals eat smaller animals like a whole chain like – fish eat the particles in the water, the plankton. The plankton go to the fish, the fish go to the people. What else?

S$_3$: The sun starts out – feeds the algae and the plankton eat the algae and the uh, the little tiny, the sardines eat the algae, too, and the fish eat the sardines ...

S$_1$: Okay, so you're not only describing a chain, you're describing a web.

S$_2$: *(Question/clarification)* What's a web, and what's a chain?

S$_1$: Okay, if you look at the picture there [refers to his book], you've got the decomposer returning food to the soil. The plant uses that, that plant may be eaten by, if you look at the arrows, by the rabbit or the squirrel. Okay, then the rabbit might be eaten by the hawk – and the rabbit might be eaten by the fox. So, a web – well, the rabbit could be eaten by the fox, too, but webs show all the different possibilities. More than one animal or plant involved.

S$_1$: *(Question)* What does a food chain look like, what does a food web look like?

S$_5$: Like a spider's web when you get all done with it.

S$_1$: *(Clarification)* Is that true, a food chain looks like a web?

S$_5$: *(Clarification)* Could somebody clarify the difference between a food chain and a food web? Are they two ways of describing the same thing?

S$_2$: Chains like, they're short – like the sun and the corn and then the animal. The web'll go on and on.

S$_5$: (Interrupting) It would be okay if we disrupted the chain at the very beginning because that would be easier to fix. If they disrupted the food chain at the end, then they'd have to fix lots of things. If they did it at the very beginning ...

S$_1$: Doesn't make a difference. If you disrupt it at the end, you won't have to fix much.

S$_1$: Then you gotta change the rest that's behind it.

S$_5$: Then you have to fix everything before it.

S$_2$: (S$_2$ gets the point). It doesn't make a difference, it's a chain, you can start in the middle, at the end. Whatever.

S$_5$: (S$_5$ gets the point). Oh, I see, it doesn't matter. If you just start something in the middle, now it goes down, and it'll disrupt something else, it'll disrupt the grass. Then that would go down the chain, disrupt that, and then that would come back up, through the fish, through the animals that eat the fish, and then through the animals that ...

S$_3$: It's a mess.

Three months later

S$_1$: *(Question)* Why do scientists think most of the sea otters will die?

S$_2$: Because they live, see, there! mostly in that section. So when the oil gets on their fur, they'll sink or get too cold. And it gets in their stomachs where they try to lick themselves clean – or drown or something.

S$_3$: We're missing the boring old chain stuff.

S$_1$: We're getting there.

S$_4$: *(Explanation)* Oil kills otters, otters eat sea urchins, sea urchins eat kelp. Kelp keeps everyone happy. Take out otters, and you got one of those broken links. Too many of some – not enough of another.

S$_2$: Another problem, it says here, is the oil on top of the water makes it dark. It's dark, and the sun can't get in so it doesn't grow. – What doesn't grow?

S$_2$: The plankton, so the shrimp's not fed and the tuna's not fed, cause it eats the shrimp, and so on in a circle – or a web?

Table 2. Students discussing adaptation over time

S_3:	*(Question)* Why did the moths change color?
S_1:	Because of the factory smoke
S_3:	*(Question)* Did they just change?
S_5:	Some did, some didn't.
T:	*(Clarification)* Do you mean a particular moth changed?
S_1:	No, no, no – they reproduced the black one.
S_4:	*(Clarification)* Like camouflage.
S_3:	No, not, not like that, not so quickly.
S_4:	Camouflage doesn't have to be fast.
S_3:	It's not just camouflage, the white ones were best at first cause they blend in. Then it got sooty, and slowly, slowly, there got to be more black ones cause they're the survivors now cause they blend in to the soot.
S_4:	But the moths don't change color after they've been hatched.
S_4:	*(Clarification)* I'm still not sure, were the white ones born white and then went black?
S_3:	No, remember the 2000 rats [reference to thought experiment from previous material] – lots of white and few blacks. As it got darker, whites were spotted and eaten so they couldn't reproduce. Black ones survived and got to be many, and they had black ones like themselves.

group of students is trying to sort out the actual mechanism of the Moths of Manchester adaptation. We would not claim that these children fully understand the biological mechanisms in question, but we would argue that they are identifying and grappling with the central problems.

Scientific Misconceptions

Not all the news was good news, however. We saw many examples of causal reasoning that reflect common fallacies and even scientific misconceptions. Tautology was popular. For example, children argue that otters sink because of their lack of buoyancy, without understanding what buoyancy means. More troubling was the introduction of the notion of intent, leading to a form of teleological reasoning [von Wright, 1971], ' ... the chameleon changes color any time it wants to really', and even the premise that black moths of Manchester seek out other black moths *in order* to have black babies and survive. Teleological reasoning about biological systems, however, is by no means restricted to children or non-scientists [Mayr, 1982].

And even more troublesome is the fact that many of our children 'progressed' from having no causal theory of events to espousing something akin to naive Lamarckian theory that acquired traits are inheritable, expressing beliefs such as: 'Animals needed to run fast for food so they practiced and got strong muscles, and their babies got those strong muscles too'. Such beliefs are very similar to the misconceptions college students have when entering biology courses [Bishop and Anderson, in press]. This finding raises several interesting questions: (1) Is it possible to delineate in detail the child's theory [Carey, 1985; Springer and Keil, 1989] and test it for robustness and consistency? (2) Is it better to hold an incorrect belief or no belief at all? (3) Can children correct their own misconceptions, or is this the place for more adult guidance?

Controversy exists over whether and how one can induce conceptual change in naive theories. The 10-year-old knows more about the concept 'living thing' than the 6-year-old [Carey, 1985], but we don't know why, or what causes the change. Educators demonstrate that exposure to a course in biology does little to change student beliefs [Bishop and Anderson, in press], but such courses are not usually designed to challenge specific mis-conceptions directly. There has been little systematic study of microgenetic learning in which children or adults are systematically faced with repeated exceptions to their own theories over extended periods of time (although see Schauble and Glaser, this volume).

Writing Examples

Over time writing samples revealed increasingly sophisticated use of argument structure, compare-and-contrast modes, and hierarchical struc-turing of content. Students progressed from producing a book that con-tained a perfectly linear structure of 22 paragraphs about 22 animals to books with a recognizable and complex hierarchical organization. By the end of the year, the best class books contained three types of organization – a hierarchy, a compare-and-contrast section, and an exemplar-based sec-tion. This mixed model is difficult for even college students to handle. These are our very best examples; not all students showed such progress. But, comparing the microgenetic change over a year with existing cross-age norms for writing, we estimate that the best students progressed from poor elementary school level to a level more typical of young adults.

Not all students were capable of such sophistication, of course, but most showed progress. The most dramatic progress came from the initially weaker writers. Consider just one example. Tom, a learning disabled sixth-grade 11-year-old reading at the second-grade level, initially spent the lion's share of his effort on graphics and had to be 'persuaded' to provide any text at all; this he 'borrowed' from a book. He refused to provide an independent handwritten sample, and both teacher and student agreed that he 'couldn't write'. At the end of the year, he was asked to design an animal on Hypercard that would be well-adapted to a certain habitat, in this case a swamp. Tom showed no hesitation in attacking this problem, even though strange adults (the authors) were watching him. He began with his favorite, graphics, drawing a splendid creature, but then he calmly added 'created' text:

(My animal eats) Most insects some small fish and a canal rat her and thereand some crafish There are small spikes all over the body and 4 long poison stingers on it tail that they are amun to so when they eat it they do not get poisined like there prey. It has a very strong noise and very sharp eye sight. It doesn't depend on other animals because its mean.

(It defends itself) There are small spikes all over the body and 4 long poison stingers on it tail that they are amun to so when they eat it they do not poisined like there pray.It has a very strong noise and very sharp eye sight. Yes they are very aggersive if you bother it would try very hard to hurt you.

On the average the female will have about 60 babys a year. they are bord under ground and the mother will get as many worms as possable.

If not for the very strange way of protection prey coule wipe out the whole litter in one atack. this strang way of proction is when they are born they do not have legs yet and it has allmost the exact pattern of a full groun corba.

This text took about ½ hour to complete. The spelling and punctuation are weak, but Tom introduced several sophisticated biological themes. For example, he incorporated the notion of poisoned spikes to which the host is immune (amun), and mimicry – the litter have no legs and look like full-grown (groun) cobras (corba), thus mimicking dangerous snakes for protection.

A Context by Any Other Name

The original reciprocal teaching method achieved success at getting poorly performing students to strive for meaning. The simple extension of this work, asking students to read texts focused on recurrent themes led to significant increases in the use of analogy and cross reference. Having students generate their own learning materials led to activities that promote deeper understanding in the search for coherent causal explanations.

Students seeking an encompassing explanation to support facts create an active learning environment for themselves that is quite different from the passive reception of assigned knowledge that too often dominates classroom interactions. Involved students brought their own outside material to the classroom – books, newspaper articles, and reports from television news. Students felt a sense of ownership over the knowledge they were acquiring. They formed a culture of learning [Brown et al., 1989], where reading, writing and thinking took place in the service of a recognized, reasonable goal – learning and helping others learn about a topic that deeply concerned them.

A Community of Learning

Within these communities of learning, students served as cognitive apprentices [Collins et al., 1989] to the adults present and to each other. Expertise did not rest with a single authority figure, the teacher; it was distributed throughout the classroom. The teacher was not a domain-area specialist. Often she did not know the answer to questions and therefore provided useful modeling of 'how to find out'. The adults had varied computer skills, ranging from essentially none to M.A. level proficiency. Similarly, individual children 'majored' in various aspects of the curriculum. Some, like Tom, became computer graphics experts, some devoted considerable time to publishing, progressing from simple aspects of word processing to quite sophisticated control of PageMaker, a desktop publishing package. Others became expert in the predicaments of various endangered species. Children readily recognized expertise and sought help from others more expert than they in some aspect of the work.

But what were the students apprenticed to? Certainly not biology. Few if any of these students are likely to go on to be professional biologists, and the teachers and researchers were not biologists either. We argue that the students were *apprentice learners,* acquiring the skills of independent and collaborative research. The collaborative setting forced the students to engage in reasoning activities overtly, so that many role models of thinking emerged [Brown and Palincsar, 1989]. We argue that with repeated experience explaining and arguing, justifying claims with evidence, etc., students will eventually come to adopt these critical thinking strategies as part of their personal repertoire of ways of knowing.

These collaborative learning classrooms diverge from traditional elementary school classes. In 'reading group', teachers assign the text and dole reading out in small pieces, and students have no right to put the task aside. This is in sharp contrast to how literate events evolved and are maintained in the real world. So too this practice is in contrast to our learning environment, where children write the texts, working at their own pace, with extended involvement in personally chosen projects. Another strange aspect of reading lessons is that students read in order to prove to the teacher that they have read and to answer questions posed by the teacher, who, clearly, already knows the answer. The teacher is also the primary consumer of any written products. But in our classroom, students answer their own questions and are accountable for the quality of the questions asked. Teachers do not always know the right answer.

Students read in order to communicate, teach, write, persuade, and understand. The goal is reading, writing, and thinking, in the service of learning about something. Teaching is on a need-to-know basis, with experts (be they children or adults) acting as facilitators. Student expertise is fostered and valued by the community. A community of discussion is created with distributed expertise. This change from traditional teaching and learning practices results in significant improvements both in the students' thinking skills and in the domain-specific knowledge about which they are reasoning.

Acknowledgements

A more detailed version of this report, containing transcripts and illustrations of the students' writing can be obtained from the authors. This research was supported by a grant from the J.S. McDonnell Foundation and the Evelyn Lois Corey Fellowship in Instructional Science to A.L.B. We would like to thank Anne Slattery, Carole Fine, Eric Buhs, and Susan Ravlin for their work on this project, and Marion Heal for her endless patience transcribing the discussions. We would also like to thank Dr. Donald Holste, Associate Superintendent of Urbana School District No. 116, and Dick Sturgeon, Principal of the Thomas Paine School in Urbana, Illinois for their enthusiastic support of this project. We would also like to acknowledge the considerable help of Patsy Pratt, Mary Rogers, and Jim Zimmerman, classroom teachers at Thomas Paine. Without their support, patience, enthusiasm, and tolerance for occasional chaos, this work would not have been possible. Finally, of course, thanks to the fifth and sixth graders at Thomas Paine, our collaborators in the community of learning. A version of this paper was presented at the annual meeting of the American Educational Research Association, San Francisco, 1989, and as the Presidential Address to Division 7 of the American Psychological Association, New Orleans, 1989.

References

Aronson, E. (1978). *The jigsaw classroom.* Beverly Hills: Sage.

Bereiter, C., & Scardamalia, M. (1989). Intentional learning as a goal of instruction. In L. B. Resnick (Ed.), *Knowing, learning, and instruction: Essays in honor of Robert Glaser* (pp. 361–392). Hillsdale NJ: Erlbaum.

Bishop, B.A., & Anderson, C.W. (in press). Student conceptions of natural selection and its role in education. *Journal of Research on Science Teaching.*

Brown, A.L. (1980). Metacognitive development and reading. In R.J. Spiro, B. C. Bruce, & W.F. Brewer (Eds.), *Theoretical issues in reading comprehension* (pp. 453–481). Hillsdale NJ: Erlbaum.

Brown, A.L. (1988). Motivation to learn and understand: On taking charge of one's own learning. *Cognition and Instruction, 5,* 311–321.

Brown, A.L., Bransford, J.D., Ferrara, R.A., & Campione, J.C. (1983). Learning, remembering, and understanding. In P.H. Mussen (Series ed.), J.H. Flavell & E.M. Markman (Vol. eds.), *Handbook of child psychology: Vol. 3. Cognitive development* (pp. 515–529). (4th ed.). New York: Wiley.

Brown, A.L., Campione, J.C., Reeve, R.A., Ferrara, R.A., & Palincsar, A.S. (in press). Interactive learning, individual understanding: The case of reading and mathematics. In L.T. Landsmann (Ed.), *Culture, schooling and psychological development.* Hillsdale NJ: Erlbaum.

Brown, A.L., & Palincsar, A.S. (1989). Guided cooperative learning and individual knowledge acquisition. In L.B. Resnick (Ed.), *Knowing, learning, and instruction: Essays in honor of Robert Glaser* (pp. 393–451). Hillsdale NJ: Erlbaum.

Brown, J.S., Collins, A., & Duguid, P. (1989). Situated cognition and the culture of learning. *Educational Researcher, 18,* 32–42.

Carey, S. (1985). *Conceptual change in childhood.* Cambridge MA: Bradford Books, MIT Press.

Collins, A., Brown, J.S., & Newman, S. (1989). Cognitive apprenticeship: Teaching the crafts of reading, writing and mathematics. In L.B. Resnick (Ed.), *Knowing, learning, and instruction: Essays in honor of Robert Glaser* (pp. 453–494). Hillsdale NJ: Erlbaum.

Collins, A., Warnock, E., Aiello, N., & Miller, M. (1975). Reasoning from incomplete knowledge. In D.G. Bobrow & A. Collins (Eds.), *Representation and understanding: Studies in cognitive science* (pp. 383–415). New York: Academic Press.

Feuerstein, R. (1980). *Instrumental enrichment: An intervention program for cognitive modifiability.* Baltimore: University Park Press.

Glaser, R. (1984). Education and thinking: The role of knowledge. *American Psychologist, 39,* 93–104.

Mayr, E. (1982). *The growth of biological thought.* Cambridge MA: Harvard University Press.

Miller, G.A. (1988). The challenge of universal literacy. *Science, 241,* 1293–1299.

Polya, G. (1973). *How to solve it: A new aspect of mathematical method* (2nd ed.). Princeton: Princeton University Press.

Resnick, L.B. (1987). *Education and learning to think.* Washington: National Academy Press.

Resnick, D.P., & Resnick, L.B. (1977). The nature of literacy: An historical exploration. *Harvard Educational Review, 48,* 370–385.

Schoenfeld, A.H. (1985). *Mathematical problem solving.* New York: Academic Press.

Springer, K., & Keil, F.C. (1989). On the development of biologically specific beliefs: The case of inheritance. *Child Development, 60,* 637–648.

Toulmin, S. (1958). *The uses of argument.* Cambridge: Cambridge University Press.

Von Wright, G.H. (1971). *Explanation and understanding.* Ithaca NY: Cornell University Press.

Vygotsky, L.S. (1978). *Mind in society: The development of higher psychological processes.* (M. Cole, V. John-Steiner, S. Scribner, & E. Souberman, Eds. and Trans.). Cambridge MA: Harvard University Press.

Whitehead, A.N. (1916). *The aims of education.* Address to the British Mathematical Society, Manchester, England.

Subject Index